# JOURNEYING ALONE, JOURNEYING STRONG:

## NAVIGATING AGING ALONE WITHOUT CHILDREN

*Self-Help Guide to Finding Inner Strength, Peace, Joy & Fulfillment in Childless Aging*

## Chrío Zoë

limited to, errors, omissions, or inaccuracies. either directly or indirectly.

This book is copyright protected. It is only for personal use. You cannot amend, distribute, sell, use, quote or paraphrase any part, or the content within this book, without the consent of the author or publisher.

Disclaimer Notice:

Please note the information contained within this document is for educational and entertainment purposes only. All effort has been executed to present accurate, up to date, reliable, complete information. No warranties of any kind are declared or implied. Readers acknowledge that the author is not engaged in the rendering of legal, financial, medical or professional advice. The content within this book has been derived from various sources. Please consult a licensed professional before attempting any techniques outlined in this book. Book

First edition

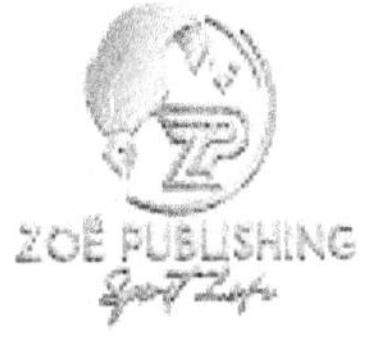

# ACKNOWLEDGEMENT

Writing this book has been a labor and a journey that I couldn't have undertaken without the incredible support and encouragement of many individuals. I am profoundly grateful to all those who have played a part in bringing this project to fruition.

I would like to thank each person who was instrumental in shaping my path to writing this manuscript. My sincerest appreciation goes to the countless friends and family who graciously gave me space and time to make this book become a reality.

First and foremost, I want to express my deepest gratitude to my family whose unwavering belief in me and constant encouragement have been my driving force. Your love and support have sustained me through the challenges of this creative process. I give honor to my late parents, Stephen and Pearl, whose unwavering belief has been the catalyst to propel me in this journey. Their constant encouragement and unconditional love have been my strength to pursue this endeavor. I say thank you to my siblings Michael, Anthony, Pauline and Sharon who have now passed on but are the silent voices that ignited me to write this book. Through their life, in their own small contributing way, I have come to realize that this journey we call life is valuable and how we start the journey does not dictate how we finish it.

I would like to thank all of my mentors and teachers who helped me by sharing their invaluable knowledge base with me, as they guided me from a place of knowing in shaping my ideas and refining my writing. I cherish your warm guidance, encouragement, and belief in me, and my potential and I can attest to the fact that it has been transformative. I am sincerely hoping that this book will serve as a helpful resource and companion guide on my readers' journey toward self-improvement, empowerment, and fulfillment.

I'd also like to thank the team at AIA and Publishing Services for their dedication and hard work in bringing this book to life. Your expertise coaching and guidance in outlining, design, formatting, and marketing have been pivotal in turning my manuscript into a polished publication.

Additionally, I am grateful to my dear friends, who provided much-needed moral support and encouragement during the writing process. I am forever grateful for your influence and for your push to encourage me into what you believe I could be. Thank you all for the guidance and the wisdom you shared with me as I stumbled along my sometimes-rocky road of personal growth and self-discovery. I extend my heartfelt appreciation to my friends and colleagues who provided valuable feedback, engaged in insightful discussions, and cheered me on during moments of doubt. Your enthusiasm has been contagious and uplifting.

Finally, I want to acknowledge my readers—those who will engage with this book. Your curiosity and interest in my ideas fuel my passion for writing, and I hope this book resonates with you in meaningful ways. In writing this book, I've come to realize that the journey is made sweeter by the presence of supportive souls. To all those I've mentioned and to anyone whose name might have been inadvertently omitted, please know that your impact has been immeasurable.

To all of you, your enthusiasm, engagement, and support to me have been more than appreciated. Let me end by saying once again to my readers that I applaud you for buying this book to enhance and empower your personal development. I trust that this book will meet your desire.

With heartfelt thanks,

**Chrío Zoë**

# Contents

# INTRODUCTION

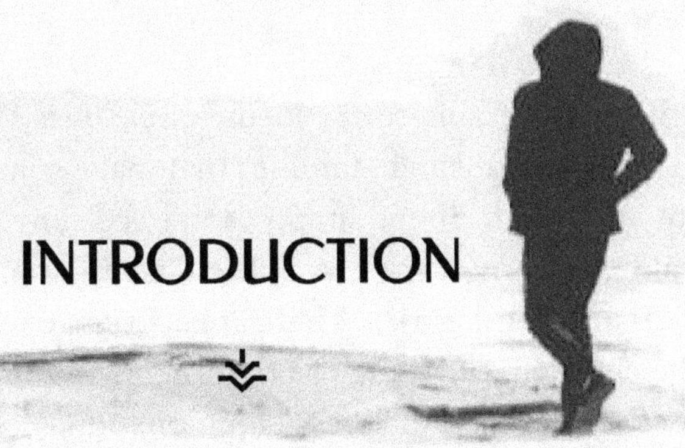

Eric and Vera were entering their 50s and past the age when they could have children. It was only then that they realized that they had a lot to do in order to plan the rest of their lives. They had lots of questions that needed answers. Some of their concerns were personal: How could they maintain their health? Where would they live? What did they need to do to ensure their retirement? Others were related to their childless state: How would they manage in their old age? Who would inherit their assets? They were excited about the prospect of moving into their golden years and satisfied with their decision not to have children. But they still needed advice and encouragement.

Lots of people are in the same boat as Eric and Vera. In fact, "Of the 92.2 million adults ages 55 and older in 2018, 15.2 million (16.5%) are childless." Also, "childlessness is more common among the younger cohort of older adults. This suggests that childless adults will make up an even greater share of the older adult population in the future" (U.S. Census Bureau, 2021).

Is that your situation? Take comfort in the fact that you're part of a trend that is growing with each passing year. People are deciding not to have children for any number of reasons. Some are worried about the state of the world and are reluctant to bring children into all that uncertainty.

Others aren't able to for medical reasons. There are health conditions that run in families that make some people decide not to risk it. Some simply don't feel any desire to have children. Many of these people enjoy children; they just don't want any of their own. There are also some who simply don't like children, as strange as that seems to the people who do have children. All these opinions and choices deserve understanding and respect.

After all, there are advantages to not having children as you grow older. You have more freedom to travel or pursue your passions. You have more resources to spend or invest in ways that bring you satisfaction. You gain the ability to concentrate more intently on your career. You have more time to yourself or to spend with a spouse or partner. You get to avoid PTA meetings, chauffeuring kids to soccer practice, and spending your time worrying about how the children will grow up.

Not having children can be difficult emotionally, though. You may have confused feelings about being a senior with no kids. You may feel lonely and isolated. You might have concerns about aging alone. You could be feeling the weight of society's judgments of your child-free state. Additionally, all the decisions you need to make might be confusing to you. Those feelings are normal and nothing to be ashamed of.

You can take heart from the example of others who are in your situation and have found satisfaction. Iconic singer and philanthropist Dolly Parton and her husband, who have been married for over 50 years, don't have children. Because of her endometriosis and the pressures of her busy career, they were never able to have a child. She has channeled her maternal feelings into improving the lives of others' children, writing songs that validate them, and donating millions of books to children through her Imagination Library (Natale, 2021).

Renowned actor Christopher Walken and his wife have been married for decades but have no children. "I do like to work as much as I can because I don't have children, and I'm glad I don't have children." It's not that he doesn't like children: "I have two brothers, and they have plenty of children," he says, but it's just that it's not for him. "They come to my house, and I am always very glad when they leave" (Adegoke, 2022).

Oprah Winfrey, Helen Mirren, Ellen DeGeneres, Margaret Cho, Keanu Reeves, Stevie Nicks, Ricky Gervais, and Sandra Oh are all child-free, too. They cite their careers, their inability to conceive, their satisfaction with being aunts and uncles, or their personal choices for their decisions. Their choices may not be the ones that most people make, but they're still valid and right for them. They've been more than able to live full, interesting, and successful lives—and so can you!

## Your Journey

Life is a journey made up of your choices. As you grow older, you have a chance to reflect on your choices and celebrate them. And you have a chance to make more choices about the rest of your life. I'm here to help with that!

Think of this book as a map to guide you on your journey. Here, you can find validation and advice to steer you over the rough spots and make that journey an enjoyable and satisfying one. Here, you'll find stories of people just like you—seniors who are living child-free. You'll also find whole chapters about the things that matter most to you. Within its pages, I'll answer your questions and offer suggestions to ease your way.

From thorny financial decisions to suggestions about diet and exercise, from building resilience to determining the legacy you will leave for the world, I'll help you untangle the many challenges you face. I know that you can face and conquer them. You'll reap the benefits of my empathy for you as a child-free senior and my years of experience and research. Together, we can chart your future and make your journey easier and more fulfilling!

Along the way, you'll discover how terrific your life really is. You can reflect on your life and recognize the freedom that you have. You can find out how to reach out and make yourself part of a vibrant, supportive community. You'll experience ways to achieve the personal growth that you so richly deserve. Moving into the next stage of your journey will be an exploration of possibilities and opportunities. Your advantages of freedom and wisdom are bringing you into the future with the tools you need to thrive.

Rest assured that after reading this book, you'll treasure your life as a child-free senior and embrace the freedoms and joys that are available to you.

The journey awaits. Let's get started!

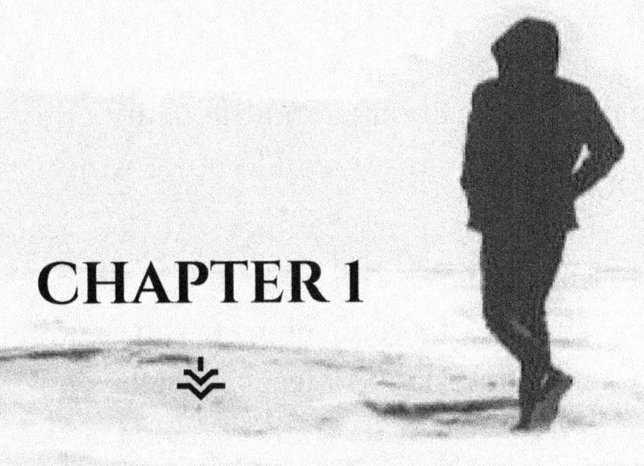

# CHAPTER 1

## THE ROAD NOT TAKEN

*Two roads diverged in a wood, and I—I took the one less traveled by, And that has made all the difference.*

—Robert Frost, "The Road Not Taken"

Robert Frost was talking about making choices. His poem clearly states that our choices are between the road that most people travel and the other one—the path that not as many people choose. And he implies that following the road that is not selected as often is preferable, at least for the narrator. The poem was written many years ago, but nowadays, we see it as an invitation to choose the road not taken—the one that leads to an unknown destination.

Throughout your life, you make choices. You decide whether to go to college and, if so, which one to choose. You may choose to share your life with another person or to remain single. You could decide that you value making money or that you intend to make the world a better place.

Each of these choices and the many others that life presents to you shape your life and your destiny.

One of the most important decisions you can make is whether to have children. If you do, you are traveling the road that most people choose. But if you live child-free, you are choosing the road less traveled. That choice comes with repercussions throughout your life. It affects how you live, what you enjoy, what struggles you have, and how you meet them.

Let's take a look at some people who took the road less traveled.

## Embracing the Path of Aging Without Children

Mary, Jo, and Jim decided not to have children. They were worried about the state of the world that they would be bringing a child into, and they had health conditions they were reluctant to pass on. They didn't regret their decision. They felt it was the right choice for them. As they reached their 50s, they enjoyed the things that a child-free life meant for them. Jim and Mary Jo remodeled their house, traveled to Scotland, and even made trips to Disney World, where they enjoyed Epcot's Wine and Food Festival without worrying about how to entertain any kids. They were occasionally bothered by friends and relatives who questioned their decision and called them selfish, but they shrugged off the comments. They were happy with their decision.

Nancy and Martin were never able to conceive a child. They went through endless rounds of infertility treatments, including in vitro fertilization, but nothing worked. Once, Nancy thought she was pregnant and rejoiced, but it turned out to be either a simple missed period or a very early miscarriage. The couple was devastated. They wouldn't consider adoption, as they desperately wanted a child that was biologically theirs. As Nancy reached the end of her childbearing years, they acknowledged the fact that they would remain childless. Nancy chose to take a job at a daycare center, which allowed her to interact with young children even though she would never have any of her own.

Anne kept postponing having a child as she pursued her career as a doctor. Working long hours and plagued by stress, she concentrated on building a life for herself. She eventually got a position in the obstetrics department of a hospital in a big city. Anne found that she enjoyed helping others bring new life into the world but realized that having a child was not for her. As a single woman, she knew that her busy career and not having a partner would have made it difficult to care for a child. When she retired, Anne surrounded herself with a circle of close friends. She was satisfied that she had made a good life for herself.

Kim and Jean wanted to adopt a child, but adoption agencies refused to even consider placing a child with a gay couple. They lobbied and worked to change the adoption regulations in their state but had no luck. The couple considered having a child via a surrogate mother but had qualms about the ethics and expense of it. As they aged, Kim and Jean worried about having no one to care for them when they became unable to care for themselves the way they had to care for their parents. Wanting to prepare for the future, they wondered whom they would name as their healthcare proxy and whom to name as their heirs.

Stu and Stephanie had a much-wanted daughter, Victoria, whom they loved unconditionally. When Veronica was 16 and trying out her new driver's license, though, her car was broadsided by a pickup truck. She lingered for a week and then died. Stephanie grieved for years, and Stu never felt the time was right to discuss having another child. The possibility became more and more remote until there was no chance left. They did not choose their childless state, but they chose how they dealt with the aftermath of the tragedy.

Each of these people remained childless as they grew older. The reasons may have been varied, but the result was the same in all their cases. Some found their lack of children tragic, while others enjoyed their child-free lives. But all of them faced the same reality—entering their later years without children. And each made a choice somehow not to pursue the path of having children.

## Your Life Choices Are Valid

Your situation may resemble one of the ones I've shared. It's increasingly common for people to remain childless throughout their lives. Despite the emphasis that modern society places on motherhood and idealizes having children, "44 percent of non-parents ages 18 to 49 say it is not too likely or not at all likely that they will have children someday" (Stein, 2023). The reasons they give are many: financial, societal, lifestyle, and other concerns. Whatever circumstances have resulted in you being a non-parent, you live every day with your status in life. It's best if you recognize it as a good option for you.

The trend of childless adults is increasing—but it's not just trendy. It's a valid life choice. You may have chosen not to have children because of your career or because a partner doesn't want them. You could have postponed having a child until it's no longer an option. You may be concerned about overpopulation or genetic issues.

The thing to know is that whatever your reason for being childless, it's a valid one. You don't have to be ashamed of not joining the ranks of motherhood or fatherhood. If you experience pushback about your choices, know that many people who do have children have mixed feelings about being a parent. Perhaps they had children too young or had more children than they could support. They may reflect on their missed opportunities. Their children may not have brought them the joy they expected.

Some people believe that the increase in child-free living has increased because of women's growing empowerment, educational choices, and job opportunities. Some attribute it to the fact that the "nuclear family" of married parents with 2.5 kids is becoming more of a rarity. And while women are now expected to "have it all"—motherhood and a fulfilling career—more and more women are finding that expectation to be impossible. Single parenthood, though it's become more common, presents even more challenges. Many people simply decide to opt-out.

The bottom line is that you don't have to have a child to be happy and fulfilled. There are so many other ways of living that don't involve children, and they are not lesser or invalid. Even people who are not childless by choice can learn to embrace their status and discover the many ways they can still find satisfaction.

And there are many ways to find that satisfaction. Throughout this book, I'll explore with you the possibilities of child-free living.

## Your Future and Your Life Without Children

As you get older, your world changes. The things you valued as a young adult may no longer seem important. Your increasing maturity brings new insights. You grow more reflective about your life. And you think about what's yet to come. Just because you're aging, your life is far from over.

Nowadays, there's no one definition of what makes a family. Children are no longer a requirement for a family. A person living single and unpartnered is a family. A couple with a cat is also a family. Divorce and remarriage don't mean you aren't a family or a lesser sort of one. Seniors on their own are certainly families. People who share a house can be a family, too. People are choosing their own families and "adopting" friends as honorary uncles, sisters, and brothers. In many ways, these families are better than the traditional sort. They don't come with financial obligations. They may live far away from you and keep in close touch anyway. You don't have to entertain them on holidays, or you can if you choose to. That's the point—different types of families or how you interact with members of your birth family can be choices.

Life as a senior without children doesn't have to be the dreary, lonely existence that too many people assume it is. There are still ways to find fulfillment—it's never too late to find happiness.

## Challenges of Child-Free Living

Of course, there are challenges that come with being a child-free senior. But there are challenges that come with every lifestyle. Singles or couples who do have children can face life with insufficient resources and competing demands on their time. Their children can even grow to be disappointments to them. They may become estranged or get so involved in their own lives and families that they neglect their parents.

Still, if you haven't had children, you'll be out of step with your peers. Mathers, in particular, like to talk about their children when they get together. When they stop doing that, be prepared to talk about their grandchildren. In such a group, you may feel awkward and even tongue-tied. It's tough to change the topic when everyone else at the table already has one.

As a childless senior, you're probably independent and self-sufficient. That's usually a good thing. But if you're ill or injured, you might not have anyone who can care for you. It's not the kind of caregiving you could need later in life, but it's still significant. Even a badly sprained ankle can mean that you need someone to go to the grocery store and pharmacy for you. If you suffer a back injury, the problem is even worse. If you don't have a spouse or partner, you'll end up relying on friends or neighbors. That can be frustrating at best. When you have no children to help, a more severe injury or illness can put you in a rehab facility.

Similarly, the upkeep of your home can be a problem. If you don't have children, you'll have to power-wash the deck, prune the trees and shrubs, shovel the snow, and repair and repaint the shutters all by yourself—or spend money to have someone else take over these tasks.

Children take up a lot of time and attention. One possible consequence of not having any is that you may be left with a lot of time and nothing to fill it up with. The stereotypical childless senior is pictured as bored and lonely. That can be more true than you realize. If you don't work at finding things to do with your time (which I'll discuss in Chapter 4), you may stagnate, which isn't good for your physical or mental health.

In future chapters, I'll discuss many of the challenges that face childless seniors. You may have to find your own ways to have fun and seek fulfillment. You'll need a support system, so you'll want to learn how to build and sustain one. You'll encounter health challenges and need to find solutions that fit your lifestyle. You'll need to consider your finances and how they'll change over the years.

But those challenges don't have to fill you with fear. Your age also means that you have lots of valuable experience navigating what life throws at you. You've developed the resources you'll need to cope. You can rely on your own ingenuity and inner strength to see you through.

## Opportunities You Can Pursue

On the other hand, going through life without children has a lot of pluses. One of the most apparent is that you will have greater financial freedom. The cost of raising one child to age 17 was estimated at more than $200,000—and that was in 2015 (Das, 2019). Child care, diapers, clothing, food, education, activities, and endless other expenses certainly add up! When you don't have that $200,000+ outlay, you could buy a nicer house, travel, invest, or save.

Time is another asset that you'll have more of. Children take up a lot of their parents' time and attention. You can use that time to build a closer relationship with your spouse or partner. (You'll even have more freedom to make love when and where you want to!) And you'll avoid the exhaustion and stress that come with trying to hold down a job or pursue a career while caring for kids at the same time.

Money and time are certainly attractive aspects of a child-free life, but they aren't the only ones. Many parents find that they're not able to be "empty-nesters" because their adult children move in with them (or never move out). Often, the living arrangements demand that the parents provide a lot of financial and emotional support. It's a problem you won't have to face.

Opportunities abound in a child-free life. It's easier to move across the country to further your career. You don't have to define your identity as being a mother or father. You can have other roles that involve children, such as a favorite aunt or uncle, that don't require the same kind of time and energy investment. When you don't have children to care for, you can devote more attention to self-care and enjoy better physical and mental health. Your choices in life will expand, and you'll discover that parenthood is not the only way to have a fulfilling life.

## Reflection

Throughout this book, I'll present a series of questions for you to reflect on. You can simply think about them, of course, but you might also want to explore them through journaling. You don't need to have a formal book to journal in. You can journal on a legal pad or using your word processing program. The goal is to have a record of your thoughts that you can return to in order to see how your feelings and thoughts grow and develop. Here are some prompts to get you started:

- What emotions do I feel regarding child-free aging?
- How can I embrace the unique opportunities my choice has brought me?
- What are the best things about living child-free as a senior?
- What difficulties do I anticipate going forward?
- How can I manage those difficulties?
- What messages have I heard about not having children?
- What are my greatest strengths as a child-free senior?

## Affirmations

Affirmations are little messages you give yourself that emphasize what is right in your world, the strengths you have, and how you deal with challenges. It's often recommended that you repeat your affirmations once or twice a day. Some people write their affirmations on sticky notes and put them around the bathroom mirror, where they'll be the first thing they see in the morning and the last thing they see at night. You can also set alerts on your phone to send you affirmations throughout the day.

Affirmations work better if you say them aloud. When you hear the messages as well as think about them, they sink in more. Alternatively, you can hold an affirmation in your mind as you meditate. Here are some affirmations to start with—feel free to create your own as well and record them in your journal.

- My life choices are valid.
- I am strong enough to handle any challenges.
- I am whole and complete the way I am.
- I am proud of who I am.
- I trust myself.
- As I breathe, I release my feelings of anxiety.
- I am grateful for the blessings in my life.
- I am enough.

## Coming up Next

Together, we've been exploring the choices you have made and the choices you can make in the future. I hope you've been empowered to think of being a child-free senior as an opportunity to savor the possibilities that life holds.

In the next chapter, I'll guide you through the process of discovering your inner strength and fostering your resilience. It's the first step toward loving your child-free life!

# CHAPTER 2

⌄⌄

# RESILIENCE AND INNER STRENGTH

*A good half of the art of living is resilience.*

**–Alain de Botton**

Resilience isn't just about surviving; it's about thriving. And in the journey of aging without children, it's your superpower. Resilience involves harnessing your inner strengths and channeling your emotions in positive directions. Through resilience, you can tap your inner strengths to see you through difficult situations and challenging circumstances.

How does resilience become a superpower? First of all, it means that you can bounce back from the inevitable curve balls that life throws at you. It also means that you can persevere when you face obstacles. In addition, resilience allows you to make choices that align with your own strengths and values in order to achieve your best life.

Resilience is not something that just happens. It is forged from what you value and how you transform those values into important parts of your personality and tools to carry you through. Resilience comes from what you believe and what you value most. Resilience can be found inside yourself, not in what simply appears in your life. Your reactions help you build resilience and discover what you are capable of.

Resilience grows as you exercise your ability to make the choices that are right for you. It grows stronger when you practice it in your everyday life. For example, Janet survived a tornado that destroyed her house. Instead of giving in to helplessness and despair, she recovered her own power by facing up to what she had to do. She did what she had to do to rebuild her house and her life. She needed resilience in order to pull herself together and confront all the details that faced her—dealing with the salvage company that helped find the treasures that survived, deciphering the documents that dealt with insurance, finding a place to live during the rebuilding, selecting an architect and contractor, picking out new furniture and fixtures, and the seemingly endless decisions that appeared without warning.

None of these were things that Janet had ever had to deal with before. Despite the changes that she faced, Janet found the inner strength to make her truly resilient and guide her through her new reality. She did what she had to do. It was difficult at times, but with her strong inner resources, she got through and came out the other side with a new house and a renewed sense of her own ability to survive.

You may not ever have to face life after the devastation of a tornado. But your everyday life presents you with a series of challenges. Being childless and getting older present their own difficulties (which we'll explore more thoroughly in the rest of this book). Like Janet, you will need to find the resilience within you to navigate them.

## What Are Your Personal Strengths and Values?

Janet had to reach deep within herself to recognize the strengths that would enable her to cope. Her strengths included intelligence, problem-solving, and flexibility. She had demonstrated these strengths in many areas of her life before they came into play so dramatically. In her 60s, when the tornado changed her life, she had already succeeded in returning to college after years in the workforce. Janet coped with challenges to both her mental and physical health. And, having decided to remain childless, she had to rely mostly on her own internal resources to make it through her challenges.

Janet's values included independence and a belief in herself. These values saw her through her varied experiences with success and satisfaction.

Your strengths and values may be different from Janet's. You may find your strength in your work ethic, your courage, or your determination. Your values may include spirituality, helping others, or honesty. Together, your strengths and your values make you who you are.

You find out what your strengths are in the course of your life. Whenever you do something you never thought you could, for example, you discover your inner strengths. Your values may develop when you are young or change as you grow and mature based on your experiences.

## Identify Your Strengths and Values

Knowing your strengths and values will help you make decisions in life and feel more confident regarding your choices.

Try these ideas to get you more in touch with your inner strengths.

One thing you can do is ask other people what your strengths are. Sometimes, a trusted friend, family member, or religious advisor can see things in you that you've never considered. They can give you important feedback and even insights regarding their view of you.

Another avenue to explore is personality quizzes. Many are available online. By answering a series of questions, you can learn more about how you operate in different circumstances and how you process the information that bombards you. For example, you may find that you rely on your senses or your judgment to analyze a situation. You could discover that a particular kind of business opportunity meshes with your strengths.

Don't forget the strengths you have in different areas of life. You may have received performance reviews at work that will highlight your strengths and make you more aware of where you could stand to improve. You may find that your strengths lie in creative pursuits that you can explore further in your spare time or when you have retired.

And remember that you can find out more about your strengths by simply trying out new endeavors. Take a class in painting or writing to learn more about your capacity for creativity. Join a local pickleball team or hiking club to try out your strengths in the realm of physical activity. Join or start a book club, and you'll have the opportunity to discover your social skills and analytical abilities.

When you think about your strengths, it's only natural to consider your weaknesses as well. But remember that weaknesses can be converted into strengths. If you find that you have difficulty making up your mind, you can use a pro-and-con chart to help you determine what's best for you. If overcoming your fears isn't your strong suit, try exposing yourself to the things you fear gradually, a little bit at a time, to prove to yourself that conquering them is possible.

When it comes to your most important values, you may not even recognize what they are unless you examine them. Here's an exercise that may help.

Think about the qualities you value in yourself or others. Make a list of as many as you can think of. Do you value financial stability? Close friendships or extended family? Health and fitness?

Next, narrow down the values that matter to you to your top five. Then, weed the list down to your top three. If you can, pick one that you consider the most important in your life. If you can't, don't worry. It's pretty common to have more than one.

Explore how you demonstrate those values in your life. Try to think of specific occasions when you put them into practice. List ways you could put them into practice more often. Keep on the lookout for opportunities. For instance, if you value charity highly, look for ways you can increase your involvement with volunteer positions or fundraising for causes you believe in.

## Develop a Mindset of Resilience

Just as you can develop your weaknesses into strengths and find ways to express your values by putting them into action, you can develop your mindset so that it benefits you as you go through daily life.

What is your mindset? It's made up of the way you typically think and how you generally approach life—your thoughts and beliefs about yourself and about life in general. Do you avoid problems or address them head-on? If your mindset is one of growth, you can convert your weaknesses into strengths. If you have a fixed mindset, you tend to view problems as something you can't change. You could have a mindset that tells you that you simply aren't good at certain things, like math, or you could believe that you *can* be good at them if you are willing to work and learn.

Resilience is basically an approach to problems. If you have resilience, you face challenges with the attitude that you can conquer them. Without resilience, you are easily overwhelmed when things don't go the way you expect them to. A mindset of resilience is not something that you either have or you don't. It's something that you can strengthen and develop.

Resilience can be particularly useful in navigating a society that expects women or couples to have children. If you receive messages that you are selfish for not having children, for example, you can increase your resilience by appreciating your ability to be selfless in other ways. If your friends or family members tell you that you will regret not having children in years to come, validate the fact that you are satisfied with your choices. And if you find yourself responding to the societal expectation that children are the only way to feel fulfilled, you can express your resilience by finding fulfillment in interacting with children in other ways, such as focusing on your extended family or working for an organization that benefits children.

## Tools and Strategies

Most of us don't come with a built-in resilient mindset. How do you develop one? It can take a little work, but there are ways to foster resilience within yourself. Here are some techniques that will help:

- **Work on self-awareness**: Examine your emotions. Do setbacks devastate you? Does the thought of coping with a disaster incapacitate you? Do strong feelings cause you physical symptoms? These are signs that you don't yet have a handle on resilience. Journaling can help you surface your emotions so that you can think about them in more depth. Mindfulness techniques can also help (you'll learn about those in a future chapter). As you become more aware of what you're really feeling, you'll begin to see how resilience can help you.

- **Practice cognitive agility**: This is the ability to view yourself and your problems from a new perspective. That's one of the keys to resilience: being able to switch gears when you need to. When you encounter a problem, you can brainstorm several different ways you could react to it or solve it. Make a list of them, then review them. You may find that you have already devised a good strategy for facing problems.

- ☥ **Reinforce social connections**: When you encounter difficulties, don't forget to draw on the experiences of people around you. They're a valuable resource that you can benefit greatly from. If you haven't managed to brainstorm solutions on your own, consult a trusted friend, relative, or even a coworker to join you in the process. Two brains can be better than one!

- ☥ **Explore emotional regulation**: Once you've examined your emotions, see what you can do to control them. Foster acceptance of your feelings instead of denying them. But then work on remaining calm and collected when you feel distressed. Reflect on your emotional reactions before you go to bed so you don't overthink them while you're trying to nod off. Learn relaxation techniques that you can use to keep your brain from going into overdrive. Telling yourself that "this too shall pass" can help you keep your troubles in perspective.

- ☥ **Cultivate optimism**: It's easy to let problems overwhelm you. Believe in your own ability to devise solutions. You don't need to be relentlessly cheerful, but keep in mind that you can analyze what's happening and respond to it with a positive yet realistic attitude. Don't let yourself get swallowed up by imagining the worst that can happen in any situation. You may not think there is a bright side to every situation—sometimes there simply isn't—but there are ways to keep gloom and doom at bay. Meditation helps many people, for instance.

- ☖ **Remember your purpose:** If you're responding to a particular situation, keep your focus on that. Don't let other issues distract you. You can figure them out later when you've resolved what's bothering you right now. Above all, your purpose is to become more resilient and better able to handle what life throws at you. Keep your eyes on that prize. It will serve you well throughout your life.

- ☖ **Build up your sense of control:** There are things that are under your control and things that aren't. Be aware of the difference, and don't waste your energy attacking problems that you can't solve. Make a list of the aspects of a situation that you can control and a list of things that you can't. Concentrate on the first list. And have confidence in your ability to cope with that.

Whatever your stage in life, believe that you are capable—able to achieve a resilient mindset and take care of yourself amid difficulties. With practice, you'll find that resilience becomes your natural reaction when you need to call on your inner strengths.

## Resilience in Action

You can approach your childlessness with resilience. You can look into adoption options or pursue technological solutions if infertility is the cause of your childlessness, for example. If those don't produce results, you can use your resilient mind by taking advantage of the techniques listed above. You can deepen your relationship with your partner if there's one in your life. You can also use these strategies to guide your thinking into accepting your feelings and brainstorming other ways to experience the joy of involving yourself in the lives of nieces and nephews, mentoring a neighbor's children, or simply expanding the things that give you happiness and satisfaction in other areas of your life.

One study explored the importance of resilience in improving the quality of life for childless couples. They determined that both people in a couple showed improved quality of life when they reacted to childlessness with resilience. They analyzed their data using a resilience scale based on questions about "personal competence...and acceptance of self and life." The results showed that strengthening the positive quality of resilience deepened the positive qualities of the couple's relationship (Ha & Ban, 2020).

## Navigating Your Emotions

I've talked about the importance of being in touch with your feelings—considering your emotions—as you learn to live a full life without children, especially as you grow older. Now, it's time to take a look at those emotions and how to deal with them.

You may think that you are at the mercy of your emotions and that they can't be changed. But the reality is that you can embrace the feelings that are good for you and improve your life. You can develop the ability to dismiss unhelpful, unhealthy emotions. The resilience you've been working on is the key to either accepting your emotions as they are or not letting them rule your life, whichever you need to do.

If your childless state is involuntary, you will likely have feelings of grief and loss, compounded by emotional exhaustion. You may feel a sense of failure, whether you're a woman or a man. You may develop relationship problems or a feeling of isolation that keeps you from getting the help and understanding that you need. Of course, it's also possible that you feel a sense of relief at no longer having to undergo the rigors of medical procedures for infertility.

However, if you have chosen to remain childless, there are still emotional waters to navigate. Despite determining that not having children is the best choice for you, you may still feel a lingering sense of regret regarding that choice. This can be reinforced by messages and societal expectations that are put on you. Many people will judge you harshly or relentlessly and say, "When are you going to make me a grandmother?" or "You'll change your mind," or "Who will take care of you in your old age?" You may have unconsciously internalized the guilt that these remarks cause and need to root them out before you can be satisfied with the life you have built for yourself.

Insensitive people are everywhere. They may ask if there was a problem that prevented you from having children and offer unwanted sympathy. Unthinking, unkind people will continue this kind of thinking even when you're past childbearing age, making remarks about all the joy you've supposedly missed out on over the years. The essence of these questions is "Don't you wish now you had children?" and an assumption that you must feel a lack in your life or regret over the choice you made. Even if you do feel a twinge of regret at times, it's really no one else's business. Yet they feel entitled to question your decision and look down on you for your choice.

You may have emotions such as resentment and annoyance toward the people who make these assumptions and invade your privacy with them. You may have a feeling that societal expectations regarding motherhood and fatherhood are unfair and damaging to your mental health and happiness. It's a challenge not to let these emotions make you turn inward and doubt your choices.

On the other hand, you may feel a sense of relief or even satisfaction regarding your choices and the lifestyle you enjoy. Other people's opinions can actually remind you that you made your decision and are happy with it. You need to remind yourself that you had good reasons for choosing the path you took. You can tap into a sense of freedom and feel justified in your child-free life. You can revel in the opportunities for joy that you have and deepen your relationship with a partner—or with yourself, for that matter.

## Understanding and Self-Compassion

Throughout this chapter, I've encouraged you to recognize your inner strength and develop your resilience of mind and heart. Beyond that, though, there are things you can do for yourself that will validate the way you feel and live. Your emotions are key. Understanding the way you feel and the reasons for it is a necessary process. Once you're in better touch with your feelings, you can begin to learn how to treat yourself with not just understanding but compassion.

## Explore Your Feelings

The first step is to understand your feelings and accept them. Feelings are not good or bad; they just *are.* Of course, once you accept your emotions, you can then decide whether they serve you well or not. If they don't, you can work on shifting your attitude or getting rid of the roadblocks that have prompted your feelings. This process is not something that you do only in your "formative" years. After all, as you continue to grow in experience and wisdom, you are continually forming your inner self according to the circumstances of your life. The alternative is stagnation, which gets in the way of happiness.

In particular, it's important to understand your feelings about childlessness. These can differ based on *why* you are childless. Childlessness caused by infertility can evoke feelings of loss, sorrow, frustration, desperation, and self-blame or blame for your partner. If you're childless because of a miscarriage, your feelings may be similar, with an added layer of guilt or resentment. In either case, you may experience a sense of time slipping away from you.

If you become childless because your child dies from an accident or illness, you could experience extreme despair, profound sorrow, overwhelming helplessness, and anger directed at whoever caused the accident, the doctors, or even God. Over time, you may move on to a feeling of acceptance, especially if your faith sustains you.

Elizabeth Kubler-Ross developed the theory of the five stages of grief: denial, anger, bargaining, depression, and acceptance. Not everyone experiences all the stages in that order, but you can expect to have many or most of those feelings. You can find lots of resources, including Kubler-

Ross's writings and other books and articles that are meant to help you through the different stages. You may find that they help you understand and deal with your emotions.

If you have chosen to remain childless, however, your emotions will likely be very different. You can, of course, experience mild regret at times, as well as confusion and resentment at the messages you get from others and from society in general. But, by and large, your feelings will be positive ones. You may find relief in making your decision, happiness in considering how your life will develop according to your own needs and wants, and satisfaction in taking control of your present and future.

You could react with regret, at least at first, when you see happy families that have children, or with a desire to find another way to satisfy positive feelings you have towards other people's children—perhaps nieces and nephews, for example.

## Self-Compassion

You've probably encountered the ideas of self-esteem, self-confidence, and self-love. But there is also self-compassion, and it's a bit different from all of those. Here's a look at what they all mean.

Self-esteem means that you accept yourself the way you are and have a sense of your own worth. You respect yourself, and your view of yourself is balanced and accurate. It's a feeling based on who you are at your core. Self-confidence is more a measure of what you can do. You believe that you can accomplish what you desire. You behave calmly because you have trust in your own abilities. You're able to take on new situations with the feeling that you can succeed when you put forth your best efforts.

Self-compassion, on the other hand, means that you treat yourself with kindness. You're gentle with yourself, and don't blame yourself if you make mistakes. Mistakes are just human nature and not a reason to beat yourself up. The essence of self-compassion is that you like yourself. Practicing self-compassion means that you treat yourself the same way you would treat a dear friend. If that person was having a hard time or felt upset, you would listen to their problems, spend time with them, and perhaps distract them from their troubles by distracting them with music, a movie, or something else pleasant.

Treat yourself with the same understanding and kindness when you're having difficulties. Understand that what you're feeling is natural. Be aware of your self-talk—the messages your brain sends you about what you're doing or what's happening to you—and dismiss them if you're judging yourself unfairly. Find ways to get your mind off your troubles by practicing self-care. Above all, know that you are worthy of being treated with the same compassion that you feel for others. You may feel inadequate at times, but you rise above it instead of obsessing about it.

## Reflection

Think about the concepts covered in this chapter and ask yourself some questions about them and how they relate to you. Here are some to consider:

- 🚶 What are my inner strengths?
- 🚶 How can I put them into practice in my life?

- ☖ What can I do to strengthen my resilience?
- ☖ What are my most important values?
- ☖ How do I exhibit them in my daily interactions?
- ☖ What feelings do I have regarding being childless?
- ☖ How can I demonstrate self-compassion?

You may want to journal about these questions to help you bring your feelings and ideas to the surface. Make lists, posters, or charts that show how you feel about each. Create a mood board that expresses what you feel about the questions. Let these aids help you understand your emotions and resolve any conflicts.

## Affirmations

- ☖ My resilience is my power.
- ☖ I can bounce back from difficulties.
- ☖ I am strong enough to handle whatever happens.
- ☖ My feelings are understandable and valid.
- ☖ I am complete the way I am.
- ☖ I value myself.
- ☖ I deserve to treat myself well.

## Coming up Next

Human connections are important when you are aging without children. In Chapter 3, I'll share with you the importance of creating a supportive environment for yourself and how to do it. You will explore what it means to connect with others and how professionals can be part of your support system if you need them.

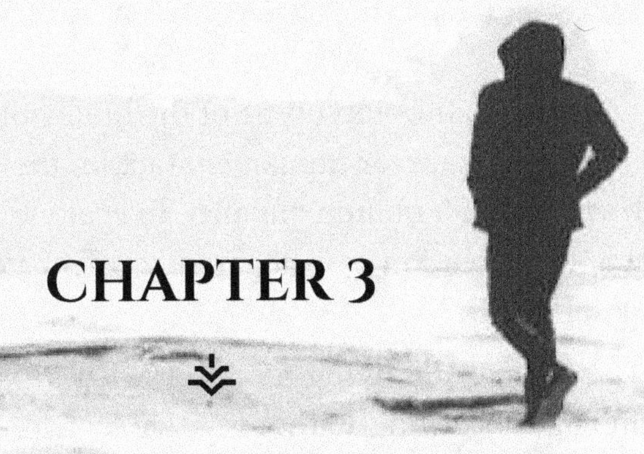

# CHAPTER 3

# BUILDING CONNECTIONS

*You can't achieve anything entirely by yourself. There's a support system that is a basic requirement of human existence. To be happy and successful on earth, you just have to have people that you rely on.*

–Michael Schur

Connection is a basic human need. No matter how self-reliant you are, you can't do without the presence of others. Think about Robinson Crusoe. The hero of Daniel Defoe's novel—who was based on a real person who was shipwrecked on a desert island—suffered terribly because he had only one other person who didn't speak his language to relieve his loneliness. By the time he was finally found, 28 years after he was stranded on the island, Crusoe even had trouble communicating with his rescuers.

Of course, you have never experienced that kind of isolation, but the isolation you do experience can have detrimental effects on your health and happiness. There's a bit of truth in the stereotype of the lonely old man or woman who is desperate for human contact. In the U.S., one-third of all seniors—14 million people—live alone (Samuels, 2023). And that isolation can negatively affect your physical and mental health.

You may be living alone or with a partner or spouse. You could be living with a relative or friends. But you need more people in your life. Not only will they help you stave off loneliness, but they will enrich your life and make you enjoy it more. They'll help you when you need help, pick you up when you're feeling down, and help you find solutions to your problems.

Rose was living alone. All her family lived hundreds of miles away and seldom visited. Her neighborhood was filled with young families just starting out, and she had little in common with them. Rose didn't drive and wasn't able to get out and about to go shopping or see a movie unless someone came by and picked her up. When her niece did call, Rose kept her on the phone as long as possible, even if they didn't have much to talk about.

Rose found a group of like-minded individuals when she joined a local church. They had a bus that picked up mostly children on Sundays, but Rose was happy to have a way to get out and among other people. She looked forward all week to Sundays. In Bible study class, she met Betty, a woman her own age who was also living alone. The two became fast friends. Rose could count on Betty for companionship. Sometimes they even went fishing together, an activity they both loved when they were young. Rose's church friends visited her when she was ill. She joined the church women's group and enjoyed participating in their holiday celebrations and dinners.

The church brought Rose the companionship and interaction she needed so much. In a sense, they were her lifeline.

## Non-Family Support Systems

What people are in your support network? Some childless seniors have other family members they can look to for support—parents, siblings, aunts and uncles, nieces and nephews, or cousins. They can provide companionship, connection, and even more material support. But not everyone has this kind of support. The people they are connected to may live many miles away and have their own lives and concerns. As difficult as it is to think about, family members may even be estranged. They're simply not available for day-to-day support or in emergencies.

Claire Samuels, a professional in the field of senior communities, notes, "Nearly one-third of all seniors live by themselves, according to the U.S. Census Bureau. That's close to 14 million seniors aging alone" (2023). Seniors in that situation have to build their own communities. It's important to expand the network of people around you if you are childless, especially if you are living alone as you age. Having human connections is vital to mental and emotional well-being. And that can be even more important than more practical forms of support.

You may think that it's simply easier to do things for yourself and that you treasure your independence, but if you have a support system, you may find that simply isn't all there is to life. Think about the physical aspects of aging. You may have to rely on a cane or a walker to get around. That's one kind of support. But other people provide a different kind of support. You need that, too.

Isolation and loneliness increased dramatically during the COVID pandemic when people were reluctant to leave their homes and have personal contact with others. Others may have been forced to work remotely, denying them many of the benefits of an in-person work environment. The results of that kind of isolation include depression, weight loss, mental decline, stress, low activity levels, and even physical problems since people weren't able to access healthcare easily.

Consider the effects of isolation on both your physical and mental or emotional health. Daily check-ins from concerned friends or neighbors can be vital lifelines if you're prone to falls. People with mental health difficulties rely on others to reach out to them at intervals. Contact with others improves their emotional health and provides a distraction from their troubles. Contact is a form of friendship that goes beyond social engagements and parties.

Yet another thing that social connections can do for you is to recommend professionals who can assist you with your needs. It's easier to find a doctor, accountant, lawyer, or church if you know someone familiar with the available options. And remember that you can do the same for them if they need help. Your own connections can be valuable to the members of your support system as well. Offering help as well as asking for it can strengthen your relationships with others.

The good news is that there are many options that can help alleviate loneliness and provide childless seniors with the benefits of connections. Friendships are the most important, including intergenerational friendships you can develop with young people. These can occur in your neighborhood or through organizations that put seniors in touch with younger people. For example, community theater groups need both younger and older actors, stagehands, costumers, and other helpers. Schools have programs that put seniors together with kids to provide oral history or learn about technological advancements. A golf foursome or tournament—or other kinds of sports groups and events—can lead to a social connection beyond the course or playing field.

Even visits from housekeepers, visiting nurses, meal delivery services, or neighbors who run errands for you bring you human contact. A casual conversation with a bus driver or store greeter can perk you right up. Many seniors look forward tremendously to these breaks from isolation. Striking up a conversation in the checkout line or doctor's waiting room requires social skills that may have grown rusty. I'm not saying that you should go on at length about your health concerns, but there are plenty of other topics to chat about. You should probably avoid politics and religion, of course, but other current events such as TV shows, movies, sports, and other entertainments that you indulge in are of interest to many different people. I've started conversations with my hairdresser simply by asking if she had seen the season finale of a TV series and what she thought would happen after the cliffhanger ending. It may not blossom into a lasting relationship, but it can definitely raise your spirits.

Remember that contact and support go both ways. Don't wait for other people to reach out to you—you can reach out to them. Reciprocity is important in friendships and other relationships. So is appreciation. Make sure the people in your support system know how much you value them and what they do for you. At the same time, it may be necessary to recognize that a support person has limits, and you should respect that. It can be tiring to listen to other people's problems every time you see or hear from them. Allow them to gracefully end a conversation, and remember that you can also set a boundary around listening to them until your eyes glaze over.

Living arrangements are something to consider when developing your social network. I'll cover this more in Chapter 6, but options like senior living communities and shared housing arrangements provide companionship and stimulation. You can even experience the rejuvenation of falling in love or finding a sexual partner. That's a good way to stave off loneliness!

## Connect Locally

Where can you find the people who will make up your support system? First, you should look around you. The people you interact with frequently can be part of your support system if you cultivate a connection with them. Neighbors, such as other people on your street or in your apartment building, can grow into a full-blown support system. Strengthen your connection with them by organizing a get-together. Consider what they're likely to respond to. A potluck dinner? A lunch date? A tea party? An outing to a museum? A bridge game or other card party? Use your imagination and leverage any interests you share. Hosting a gathering is a great way to get to know people who can grow to become part of your support system.

Professional associations are also good opportunities for getting to know others and building up your communication or business skills at the same time. Local business groups such as Rotary or Lions and fundraising groups like Friends of the Library or a hospital association always welcome new members. In addition to meeting other folks, you'll be benefiting your community—always a good way to boost your self-esteem.

There are undoubtedly plenty of opportunities in your community and activities you can join. Looking around will help you find them. For example, you can read the bulletin at your place of worship, apartment clubhouse, or gym. You can ask neighbors or coworkers what groups they belong to. When you join a group, you can assist with a membership drive, so there will be even more people you can meet!

Expand your horizons. If you have an interest or hobby you've let slide, take it up again and look for opportunities to share it with others. If you enjoy gardening, for example, you could join a gardening club, but you could also take a class in flower arranging or volunteer to work at a local arboretum. If you haven't done your favorite craft in a while, find a ceramics studio where you can create gifts for others or learn a related skill like throwing pottery.

Another place to meet new people is your public library. No longer a stuffy place where people are shushed, libraries have become a hub of activity. They host book clubs and discussion groups, civic group meetings, and events where you can read to children (and meet their parents). Speakers and local authors often come to libraries to give lectures or promote their books. Question-and-answer sessions allow people to engage with each other and with the presenters. Bookstores are good for these kinds of activities, too. They often host writers' groups where you can get feedback on your creative efforts and offer your take on others' creations.

## Connect Electronically

Don't be afraid to get online! If you're not already savvy about the internet, take a course in navigating cyberspace. Young people can be helpful guides and tutors as you explore. You don't have to learn how to program a computer (though, of course, you could), but you can learn to use some of the available software programs, such as spreadsheets to track your expenditures for tax purposes, word processors to create newsletters for the groups you've joined, and email services to keep you in contact with your friends and relatives who live just down the street or far away—even overseas. One woman I know developed a friendship with a woman in India and was able to host her when she made a trip to the U.S.

Join an online community such as Facebook or Pinterest. Within those sorts of meeting places, you will find many groups to join that explore your own interests. If you follow politics, there are many, many people and groups that communicate about developments from any point of view. There are groups for childless people and senior singles. If you are interested in humor, for example, you'll find lots of groups that delve into comedy movies or songs, as well as groups that specialize in writing newspaper columns or humorous blog posts.

Speaking of blogs, it's not hard to start one of your own. If you have tips to share about crocheting or opinions on current events, you can put them out into the electronic world and share your insights with people you don't already know. You can also make TikTok videos and post them online. You can attract a following of people who read your posts or view your content faithfully and make comments on them.

But even if the only online activity you pursue is email, you still have a valuable tool to establish connections. Email is, in many ways, better than the phone. You don't have to worry about whether your friend or relative is away from home or even asleep. Your message will be there to greet them when they finally check their email. Many people check their email several times a day, so your messages have a good chance of getting to the recipient quickly. When you receive an online message, you can think about how you want to reply before you respond. And you can send attachments, such as photos, cartoons, and links to articles from online sources, along with your emails. Online dating is also a possibility. There are dating services that specifically cater to people at your time of life.

Even if you never meet in person, you can establish important bonds with people you meet online. You'll find people who check in on you regularly—those who notice when you haven't shown up in a while. You'll have a way to contact friends who live across the country, posting pictures of your latest vacation for all to see or even your dinner out, which can start a discussion of good local restaurants or dishes to try.

## Friend to Supporter

So, by now, you have a pretty good idea of where to find friends. But how do those friends become part of your support system? What should that support system look like, and how does it function?

First, don't discount the power of simple friendship. There's nothing like a group of friends to enrich your life and give you joy. Hanging out with friends, talking to them, and making plans with them are all good in and of themselves. But if you nurture the friendship and make it deeper and more meaningful, you have the basis for a growing support system.

What makes a good support system? How can you grow your circle of friends into a true support system? For a start, don't expect any one person to be your support system all by themselves. Even a married couple needs a larger support system than just their spouse. You need someone outside the relationship. After all, you need to have someone you can turn to if you want to vent about something your partner has done!

It's not reasonable to expect any one person to be your entire support system. That's too big a burden to put on them. Even people you think of as your close friends can't always be there for you when you need them. They have their own lives and problems. If you lean on them too much, they'll burn out. Even a very devoted friend needs a break sometimes.

Having a variety of people around you is important. These people will serve different functions in your life. Maybe Tom is able to distract you when you're feeling low. You met him at the gym. Robbin is the person you can turn to with career problems. She was a coworker at your previous job. Peggy is there for deep discussions. You two went to high school together. You and Michael share confidences that go beyond the superficial. You feel comfortable with him because you know what you tell him won't go any further. Each of them is an integral part of your support system. Each nourishes you in a different way.

The heartbeat of a support system is reciprocity. They're there for you, but you're also there for them. You can't expect anyone to always be the giver. That's a recipe for burnout. Just think—even a paid caregiver is entitled to time off! If you want someone to check in on you, check in on them from time to time. Don't wait for them to invite you to a social gathering. You extend an invitation once in a while. You'll be strengthening the bond with your support system.

Another important factor is vulnerability. It's tough to open yourself up to another person, but it's the best way to grow your support system. Don't pretend that your life is perfect. No one's is. Sharing your troubles with someone else—and listening when they share theirs with you—is how you bond in a deeper, more meaningful way. Someone who opens up their real life to you is someone you care about, and vice versa.

## Support Groups and Other Options

Sometimes, support means more than just connecting with friends and neighbors, important as that is. At times, you may need professional help. Fortunately, there are sources of support out there that can help you meet your deeper needs.

Most people feel depressed or anxious at times. There's nothing really wrong. They're just having a difficult time, but it passes. If you find yourself with depression or anxiety that doesn't wear off, though, you may need to add a professional to your support system. A therapist or counselor is someone who can help you deal with what's troubling you—that's what they're trained to do. They can take over the responsibility of listening to you, connecting with you, and helping you develop strategies that will take you to a better place.

Another option is a formal support group. When you think of support groups, you may envision psychological group therapy or a 12-step group like Alcoholics Anonymous or Gamblers Anonymous. But those aren't the only kinds of support groups.

There are support groups for every stage of life and every concern. You can find groups that welcome people with medical conditions, like cancer survivors or cardiac rehab patients. But there are also groups for your stage of life or problems that you may have. If you have suffered the loss of a loved one through either divorce or death, there's a group for that. If you're single, there are meet-and-mingle groups. If you're struggling with being childless, you can find a group of individuals with the same questions and difficulties.

Support groups help because they allow you to share your troubles and thereby lessen them. You discover that you're not alone and that other people feel the same way you do. You can share strategies that help you cope and learn strategies that others have developed. You may be paired with a "sponsor" who will work with you one-on-one and be there for you if you need a friend during a particularly difficult time. Sometimes, there are speakers who have special expertise on a topic. (Support groups are also traditionally where you can find bad coffee and maybe pastries.)

## How to Find Help

Finding a support group isn't that difficult. If you do see a therapist, they can point you in the right direction. Ask them to recommend one. There may also be a group that they facilitate. Many therapists have brochures in their waiting rooms that describe recommended resources.

Self-help groups often advertise their meetings at the places that host them. If the group meets at a community center or house of worship, there will be posters that give the date and time when people gather. Then, too, you can use Google to find a support group in your area. Many national organizations have local groups they're affiliated with.

If you're nervous about going to a support group, that's only natural. You could ask a sympathetic member of your social network or support system to go with you. You may be surprised to find that there are already people you know who belong to the group.

## Reflection

Think about your current support system and brainstorm ways to expand it in the future. Explore what you need from a support system and consider who might be able to fill those roles. Ask yourself questions such as these:

- What types of support do I value most?
- What types of support do I already receive?
- What types of support do I still need?
- Who in my circle of friends can I reach out to for support?
- Are there areas of life where my needs are not being met?
- What sources of support are available in my area?
- How can I be a part of other people's support system?
- How do I give back to the people who support me?

## Affirmations

Reinforce the efforts you are making to build your support system. Acknowledge the ways you can be part of a support system for someone else.

- I can reach out to others.
- I have things to offer my friends and loved ones.
- I am able to make new friends.
- I appreciate my friends and show them how I feel.
- I am thankful for the people in my support system.
- Other people give me strength.

## Coming up Next

With a network of support in place, you're ready to explore the joys and passions that make life vibrant and exciting. In Chapter 4, I'll lead you on a journey into the world of hobbies, travel, and personal fulfillment.

# CHAPTER 4

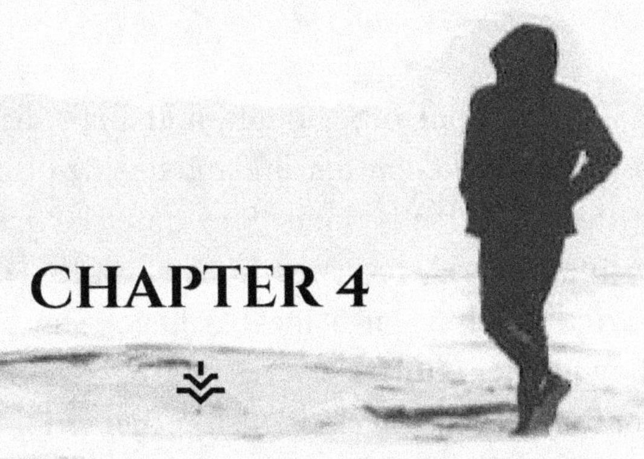

# FULFILLMENT, OPPORTUNITIES, AND YOUR JOY IN LIFE

*Life finds its purpose and fulfillment in the expansion of happiness.*

–Maharishi Mahesh Yogi

Beth was so convinced that she didn't want children that she had her tubes tied. Then she met and married a man who also didn't want children. For a while, it seemed like their lives were going great. They traveled to exotic locales and pursued hobbies, though not always the same ones. She was interested in writing. He wanted to explore flying. Eventually, they grew apart. He cheated on her, and they went through a painful divorce.

After the divorce, Beth was lonely and confused. Beth sold the house they had shared and found a small condo. She didn't rethink her desire not to have children, but she went as far as supposing that if she met a man who already had children, she might consider marrying him. But she wasn't very enthusiastic about the prospect. She definitely wanted to marry again.

Time went on, though, and Beth didn't find the right man. She looked at her life and decided that she could make a life for herself alone. She quit the job she had in the business world, returned to her first love—psychology—and started teaching at a local college. She began writing and showed her stories to friends to get advice on how to improve. She traveled with other friends and with her mother. She took up swing dancing and joined her church choir. She auditioned for and appeared in local theater productions. Before she knew it, she was living a full life without her ex-husband and without children. Beth settled into her new life and was happy.

Beth discovered that she didn't have to rely on children or the prospect of stepchildren to be satisfied. A new job and new interests kept her busy and satisfied her need for interaction and fun. Rather than wallowing in her troubles or regretting that she had decided not to have children, Beth got on with her life and found new sources of joy.

Joy is an important factor in anyone's life. It's a joy that keeps you going when parts of your life are difficult. Having a job that makes use of your talents and friends, you can share your interests with are sources of pleasure and satisfaction. Enjoying the life that you have built for yourself without children, combined with the experience you've acquired over the years, can be the catalyst for you to explore activities that you haven't indulged in lately or that you discover anew.

So, kick up your heels! Do what you've always wanted to do. Expand your horizons. You have the opportunity to fill your life with the things that make you happy. Take advantage of it! Think of your child-free life as a springboard for the exploration of your wishes and dreams or as a blank canvas ready for you to paint with all the colors of your imagination. If you seize the opportunities available to you, you'll enrich your life and keep your mind engaged with learning, travel, and social involvement.

## Pursue Your Passions

When people talk about finding their passion in life, they often mean pursuing a new vocation or getting a new job that makes use of their talents. That's happening more and more these days. The COVID pandemic allowed many people to work remotely or reconsider their job choices altogether. Some of them looked for new jobs that they could perform from the comfort of their own homes. Others decided to turn a hobby or interest, such as jewelry making or landscaping, into a business. If you do this, it should be something you are really passionate about. You know how much time and effort it takes to find a new job. Starting your own business can be even more intense. But if it's a labor of love, you will find time flying as your satisfaction increases.

Whether you're living alone, like Beth, or with a partner or spouse, think about your life up until now. What did you enjoy in the past? Even the things you remember from your childhood can provide inspiration for activities to revisit. If you liked roller skating, for example, you could rent or buy yourself a pair of skates and head out to the roller rink. If English was your favorite subject in school, you could join a book discussion group. If you have always enjoyed art, you could become a docent at a local museum or join a class to renew your love of sketching or sculpture.

There are other ways to explore your options and decide what you feel passionate about. Here are some avenues to pursue:

- Pay attention to what you enjoy talking about or teaching. Gwen found that her voice became more animated, and her interest perked right up when she talked about mystery novels with her brother-in-law, Steve, and her friend Margaret. Before long, she was writing a mystery novel of her own.

- Look at *why* you enjoy certain activities. Is it the intellectual challenge you like? Interaction with other people? A chance to express your creativity? Being outdoors? Mentoring or being mentored? Helping others? These insights can guide you in choosing a path to explore further.

- Remember the list of your most important values that you made in Chapter 2? Look for activities or jobs that align with them. If your faith is important to you, you might enjoy starting a religious study group or supporting a charitable mission. If good health is one of your priorities, you could get involved with a senior exercise program at your local continuing education program. In fact, you might end up teaching a class!

- Reach out to other people. Talk with them about their passions and how they discovered them. If someone talks about a pursuit that interests you, ask them if they would like to mentor you in that activity. Or simply ask them about joining an interest group they belong to.

🚶 Take your time. You don't have to focus on one choice right away. After taking cello lessons for a while, for example, you may find that you really don't enjoy the practice time you have to put in. Maybe you'd enjoy working at a local radio station more. Or you could switch gears entirely and take a cooking class instead.

Whatever you decide to try, keep in mind that it's not necessarily a long-term commitment. You can "shop around," trying out activities until you find what you respond most to. You can sample the possibilities that are offered as courses at a local continuing education program, senior center, or recreation center. You can invite a friend to share the experience with you or make new friends who enjoy the same things you do. You might even find a new person you can share your child-free life with!

You can even explore the more conventional definition of passion. Age isn't a barrier to sexual enjoyment anymore. In fact, not having children who might interrupt your love-making can turn out to increase your pleasure!

## Discover Hobbies

Not every interest you have has to become a passion. Sometimes, you simply want interesting activities to do when you have some time—or can make time for them. If you enjoy needlework, for example, you could try to turn crocheting into a home business. But you might enjoy it more if you simply take it at your own pace and set small goals for yourself, like creating items for a church bazaar or as holiday gifts. And speaking of needlework, the possibilities in that area are nearly endless. You may choose knitting or crochet, but you could also consider quilting, sewing, embroidery, needlepoint, or another of the fabric arts. Beth took up cross-stitch and joined a "Stitch and Bitch" sewing circle!

You can also decide whether you like that kind of interaction with other people or prefer something you can do on your own, just to relax. You can choose an activity that has a specific goal, like raising money for the library fund, or a less structured one, such as jogging just for fun. You can start small with a modest investment in model trains before you go full-tilt into building elaborate layouts for them. You could decide to take up a hobby that doesn't require much monetary investment, like power walking, or one that you can invest in, like wine tasting.

Hobbies provide many benefits. Relaxation is a good way to relieve anxiety, and crafts can develop your hand-eye coordination. You can improve your physical health with a form of exercise that appeals to you. Swimming, for example, can lower your blood pressure and help strengthen your muscles, and running releases endorphins—the "feel-good" chemicals your brain produces. You can keep your mind engaged with puzzles, reading, or discussion groups. Social engagement reduces depression, and music stimulates parts of your brain. It's hard to think of a hobby that doesn't improve life!

And if you feel that you want to share your interests, you can even consider introducing children to your favorite activity. You can get involved in children's lives without being a parent if that's something that appeals to you. You don't have to have children of your own to enjoy spending some time tutoring them, working with them on a community garden, or helping them learn a skill they need for a scout badge. You could make costumes for a school play or teach a neighbor child to play chess.

## Explore the World

Of all the possible interests and activities, perhaps the most appealing and beneficial is travel. Exploring your city, community, state, nation, or world can revitalize you, put you in contact with interesting new people, broaden your intellectual horizons, allow you to relax and enjoy yourself, or just see the sights. You can hike, boat, travel by train or plane, visit museums, see concerts and shows, explore natural wonders and national parks, go shopping or dancing, and so much more.

Dan and Ella, a childless couple in their 60s, took their "bucket list" trip to Ireland for ten days recently. They planned their trip for months, consulting guidebooks and Dan's nephew, a travel agent. They visited small towns and famous landmarks, stayed at a series of bed-and-breakfasts and nice hotels, dined on fresh seafood, and took a ferry trip to a tiny island off the coast. They took photos and posted them to social media and Ella's blog. They had indulged their love of travel many times before, taking sailing trips in the Caribbean and off the coast of Maine, touring Croatia, and relaxing in a condo just a few hours from their home. Dan and Ella credit travel with keeping their marriage and their lives fresh and interesting. Their home is filled with souvenirs, and their minds are filled with memories.

Many people think travel is best when you share it with a spouse, partner, friend, or relative. There are many exciting opportunities for groups who want to travel together and let someone else do the planning. Others prefer to travel solo and meet new people wherever they go. Each of these types of travel has something to recommend.

Traveling with another person is special. You can bond over shared experiences and have time to yourselves. You can choose your own itinerary and activities. You can plan beforehand or be more spontaneous. You'll learn more about the person you're traveling with, even if you have known each other for many years. Sharing your impressions of the places you visit can bring you closer together. Those shared experiences will enrich your lives and create memories you'll treasure for years to come.

Group travel is very attractive to many seniors. It has the benefit of letting someone else make all the arrangements and be responsible for ensuring a pleasant, enjoyable experience. It has the security of providing a tour guide to shepherd you through airports and handle any emergencies that arise. And it can be much more cost-effective than booking the trip on your own. Plus, you can find guided tours that feature a theme, such as classical music, architecture, cuisine, and other interests, as well as trips for cyclists, boaters, or hikers.

If you've been independent all your life, traveling with a group might seem like a drag. For the adventurous senior, solo travel is an option. If the freedom you get from journeying on your own is important to you—as it is for many—you can build your own adventure. Flexibility, spontaneity, and the opportunity to exercise your self-reliance are just some of the benefits. You can set your own pace and determine your own itinerary and timeline. You can change your plans easily if a new opportunity presents itself. And if your interests include meeting potential partners, there are tour companies and resorts that specialize in travel adventures for senior singles.

**Travel Tips**

Child-free seniors can make sure their travels go well by investigating their options and making some preparations.

- Airlines offer services that can help make your trip smoother and easier. You can cut down on standing in lines if you book your ticket online and print out your boarding pass before you even go to the airport. If you have a smartphone, you may not even need a paper boarding pass. If you take advantage of online booking, you can also select your seat or arrange for a special meal.

- Organizations like AARP often provide travel discounts and deals as part of their services. Airlines may also offer senior discounts, though they don't usually advertise them.

- If you have mobility challenges, airlines allow you to travel with a cane, walker, electric scooter, or even a wheelchair on board the plane. Just ask the flight attendant to store it in the plane's coat closet. You can also request someone to meet you at your gate with a motorized cart or wheelchair to get you to your next connection. Make these requests when you make your reservations.

- ⚑ You may find your trip more enjoyable if you make one location your "base of operations" and then branch out on day trips from there. That's also a reason to consider a cruise—most of your amenities and entertainment are in one place. And you'll have the opportunity to leave the ship for activities at destinations along the way.

- ⚑ You can book entrance to many attractions and activities online before you even leave home and pay for them with your credit card. This can let you "jump the line" when you get there. (You do have a credit card that gives rewards for travel, dining, and entertainment purchases, don't you?)

- ⚑ If traveling overseas causes you to worry about safety, the U.S. State Department has a website that lists travel advisories. You can also find online information about health alerts, visa requirements, and what vaccinations are required for different destinations.

- ⚑ Check with your phone carrier to learn how to make international calls or to get a temporary plan that covers them. Also, get in touch with your credit card companies. You'll need to notify them if you travel abroad so they won't question foreign charges.

## Opportunities in Your Community

You don't have to travel abroad or even far from home in order to find engagement and joy, though. There are lots of opportunities right in your own area. You can indulge your passions, explore new creative outlets, and generally have a good time. You can enrich yourself and your community at the same time!

## Activities

Every year, Tom and Leslie, senior singles, head to the Ann Arbor Arts Festival, a large local event that draws exhibitors and art-lovers from all over. In addition to paintings, drawings, and fabric arts, the festival features performing artists, such as singers and instrumental performers, costumers, acting troupes, and psychics, for a multi-day bonanza of talent. Tom, a guitarist and singer, delights in the music and often buys performers' CDs, while Leslie, who's involved in community theater, prefers the costuming and comedic actors. When they come back together after a day at the festival, they share the treasures they've found and the stories they have about their discoveries.

Most communities have arts-and-crafts fairs that may not be as elaborate as the one in Ann Arbor but are still worth your time. You can stroll among the booths, sometimes observing as the participants work on new creations and sometimes contemplating purchases of jewelry, dolls, aprons, woodworking, or tie-dyed t-shirts. If you have a creative hobby or a home business, you can also get involved as a vendor.

Other popular events include festivals that celebrate holidays with singing and crafts or ones that feature a local farm product like strawberries, popcorn, or even garlic. The many ways that they can be used are highlighted with booths selling food, including uses you've never thought of— strawberry steak sauce or popcorn-flavored cotton candy, for example.

Your community's ethnic makeup is another opportunity for fun. Local Italian, Greek, Caribbean, Polish, Jewish, or other populations present food, crafts, music, dancing, historical costumes, and cultural presentations that can occupy you for whole days or even a weekend. You can be a visitor or lend a hand in creating a celebration of your heritage!

Museums are great places for learning and fun. Art museums often have rotating exhibits as well as permanent collections, so you can enjoy them several times a year. They can also offer art lessons, such as drawing and sculpture, in which you can participate. Other museums celebrate science and natural history. Look for museums with more than exhibitions and a gift shop, though those are fun too. A natural history museum may include an IMAX theater with huge movies of animals or exploration, or it could have a planetarium to contemplate the astronomical aspects of the galaxy.

Speaking of the galaxy, many communities hold conventions that cater to a variety of interests—science fiction, gems and minerals, antiques, and Civil War re-enactors, to name a few. Many of them also feature shopping opportunities as well as the ability to mingle with other enthusiasts and noted personalities in your particular field of interest.

So, explore the attractions that are near you! Too many of us overlook what's close by when it could offer diverting and enlightening afternoons or weekends. These are opportunities that you can visit during off-hours when crowds aren't so large, and there may be a break from the heat. For instance, you could visit a museum when it opens for the day or a convention during the evening when others are settling in for family time at home.

## Volunteering

Volunteer opportunities are some of the most enriching and enjoyable for you personally as well as for your community. You can use your skills to benefit others, but you can also volunteer in ways that will develop your personal or professional skills. You can volunteer in ways that will affect your city or your environment and age groups, from seniors like yourself all the way to college students, teens, and children. Kelly, for example, works as a docent at a local arboretum to satisfy her love for nature and use her experience as a biologist. Joanne mentors young women in sales and marketing. And Michael's background in teaching and electronics helps him coach a local robotics team.

Your primary goal may be to benefit other people or your community, but you should realize that volunteering can be good for you, too. Outdoor activities can provide health benefits like increased physical fitness and lowered stress. Mental health can be improved too, by lessening your isolation, giving you an increased sense of purpose, and improving your self-esteem. Volunteering with business organizations will provide you with networking opportunities and can increase your knowledge. In general, volunteering can relieve a sense of isolation and fight depression. Plus, volunteering looks good on your resume if you are thinking of changing jobs or expanding your skill set.

Here are a few other ideas for volunteer opportunities:

- 🚶 local and national charitable organizations like food banks, Habitat for Humanity, or Meals on Wheels
- 🚶 animal shelters
- 🚶 foster grandparent programs
- 🚶 community gardens
- 🚶 a local hospice organization or a hospital
- 🚶 teaching courses for continuing education
- 🚶 political campaigns
- 🚶 libraries and literacy programs
- 🚶 neighborhood watch

## Fulfillment Through Spirituality and Mindfulness

Jack was a seeker from an early age. In his youth, he joined the seminary and dreamed of becoming a priest. But it wasn't right for him, and he left. During the years to come, he lost touch with a sense of spirituality, until a 12-step group got through to him with its concept of a "higher power." Jack began his spiritual search anew. He studied the Jewish scriptures. A woman friend introduced him to New Age religions. His job in parks and recreation made him a nature lover, and he responded to their philosophy of communicating with the natural environment. At last, in his 60s, Jack returned to his ethnic roots and began exploring the Russian Orthodox church. There, he found the spirituality he had been searching for. His quest for a tradition that he could embrace enriched his life and put him in touch with a wide variety of people who became close friends. His later years were filled with a sense of connection with other people, and the world around him, and an understanding of many faiths.

As Jack found, spirituality doesn't always mean an organized religion. It can also include personal expressions of faith, learning about and sampling from different spiritual traditions, or searching out a like-minded community where you feel welcome and comfortable. In general, religion is practiced in groups, while spirituality is more of an individual or private practice. Spirituality emphasizes a journey of discovery; religion more often centers around the worship of a deity, which can differ depending on whether you practice Christianity, Judaism, Islam, Buddhism, Shinto, Native American religion, or another tradition. Of course, there are exceptions.

Within organized religions, there is a vast difference not just between denominations and sects but also between individual spiritual communities. Some emphasize scripture study, while others have robust forms of singing and vocal prayer at worship. Many are involved in social and charitable work, like homeless outreach. Others send missionaries to work locally or in foreign countries. Finding one that provides you with a sense of the holy can be a lifelong quest that is valuable in and of itself.

## Meditation and Mindfulness

Practices such as meditation and mindfulness are also ways to get in touch with the potential within yourself. They have the added benefit of lowering stress and calming your nerves.

Meditation is easy to get started with. It doesn't require much in the way of preparation. You don't need special clothing or equipment. As long as your clothing is loose and comfortable, it will be fine. You don't have to sit cross-legged on the floor, either, though you can if you want to. All you really need is a chair to sit in that has a straight back where you are comfortable. You can use a small object, such as a flower or candle, to focus your attention, or you can simply meditate with your eyes closed.

There are many different kinds of meditation, from transcendental meditation to "moving meditations" like yoga and tai chi to Zen practices and visualization. They can help you with physical or mental health, a sense of clarity and calm, and an invigorated spirit. You can find plenty of resources online, such as videos that will demonstrate meditation practices or guide you through meditations for visualization or gratitude.

One of the basics of meditation is breathing. You pay attention to your breathing in order to center yourself in your body. Practicing different patterns of breathing will focus your attention on something other than your intrusive thoughts, as well as oxygenate your blood, body, and brain.

Mindfulness is a form of meditation that is becoming increasingly popular because it adds to so many parts of life and can be practiced at any time and in any place. Mindfulness helps you live in the moment and direct your attention closely to what you are doing in that moment. Variations of it include simply breathing mindfully or experiencing the information that your senses bring to you. Mindful breathing, mindful eating, and mindful activities are all possible.

## Reflection

In this chapter, you've been exploring what you love, what you believe in, and ways you can add joy to your life. Facing life with a sense of exploration can help you develop those sources of joy. Here are questions to consider as you think about passions, joy, and spirituality.

- What brings me the most joy in life?
- How can I incorporate that joy into my daily life?
- What are some hobbies I could rediscover?
- What place have I always wanted to travel to? Why?
- What volunteer activities can I participate in that will benefit my community?
- How do I define spirituality?
- What spiritual practices will add the most to my life?

## Affirmations

Reinforce the qualities you have that make you a vital person with many interests and abilities. How these manifest in your life is up to you!

- I am passionate about my life.
- I have many interests that bring me joy.
- I have talents to use in my community.
- I have a giving heart.
- I am brave enough to try new things.
- My spirit is strong and joyful.

## Coming up Next

You've been exploring the most rewarding things in your life. Now, you need to think about how you can ensure you have the resources to pursue them. It's time to learn all you can about the factors that enable your participation in your best possible life—security through finance and legal strategies. Don't worry! I'm here to help you!

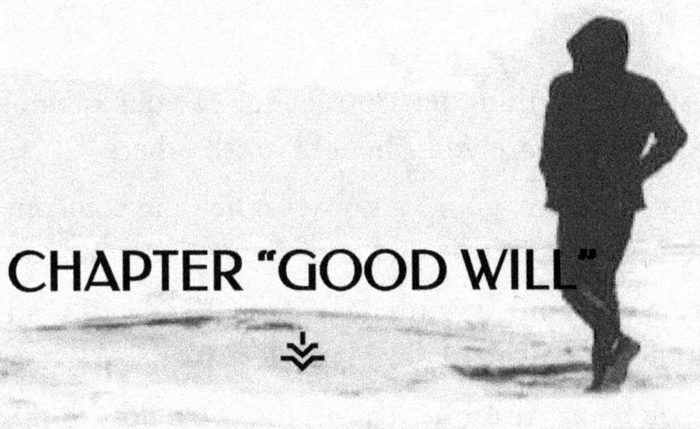

# CHAPTER "GOOD WILL"

elping others without expectation of anything in return has been proven to lead to increased happiness and satisfaction in life.

I would love to give you the chance to experience that same feeling during your reading or listening experience today...

All it takes is a few moments of your time to answer one simple question:

*Would you make a difference in the life of someone you've never met—without spending any money or seeking recognition for your good will?*

If so, I have a small request for you.

If you've found value in your reading or listening experience today, I humbly ask that you take a brief moment right now to leave an honest review of this book. It won't cost you anything but 30 seconds of your time—just a few seconds to share your thoughts with others.

Your voice can go a long way in helping someone else find the same inspiration and knowledge that you have.

Are you familiar with leaving a review for an Audible, Kindle, or e-reader book? If so, it's simple:

If you're on **Audible**: just hit the three dots in the top right of your device, click rate & review, then leave a few sentences about the book along with your star rating.

If you're reading on **Kindle** or an e-reader, simply scroll to the last page of the book and swipe up—the review should prompt from there.

If you're on a **Paperback** or any other physical format of this book, you can find the book page on Amazon (or wherever you bought this) and leave your review right there.

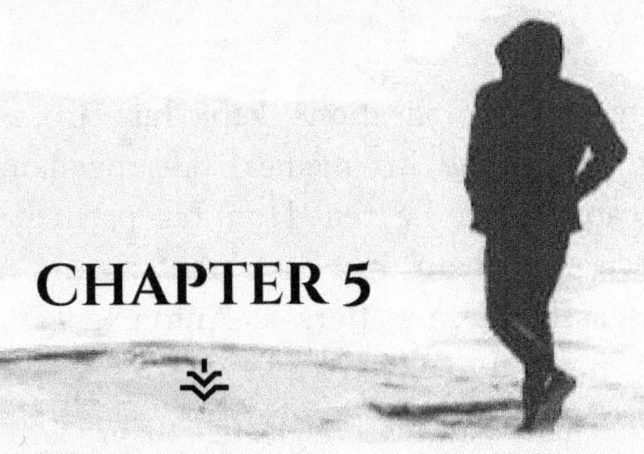

# CHAPTER 5

⍖

# LEGAL AND FINANCIAL PLANNING

*A big part of financial freedom is having you heart and mind free from worry about the what-ifs of life.*

–Suze Orman

Clark thought he had all his affairs in order, but he was mistaken. He thought he'd have enough funds to last him the rest of his life, thanks to the 401(k) plan he had at his job. He didn't realize that the contributions he'd made and the places he'd invested the funds were far from adequate. Because he thought his future was taken care of, he neglected to make any additional investments.

When he retired, Clark rapidly burned through his retirement money. By the time he was in his 70s, there was little left. Social Security wasn't much help. He was forced to downsize from a modest house to an even more modest apartment. He had to cut out the travel he loved and stop dining out so often.

Then Clark developed health problems. His heart attack put him in the hospital, and he had several stents put into his arteries. Complications kept him from returning home promptly, and his medical bills piled up. While he was incapacitated, he relied on his partner, Anton, to make decisions about his care. Anton and Clark had never discussed these matters, so Anton was at a loss about what he should do.

Clark had also neglected to prepare a will. When he passed, there wasn't much to leave for Anton. Lawyer and probate fees took up the little that was left. Clark simply hadn't made any plans for his future. His later life was a shambles, and Anton was left to deal with it.

Plenty of people are as unprepared for their future as Clark was. Did you know that 67% of Americans haven't put plans in place for financial concerns that arise at the end of their lives? According to a recent survey, "40% just haven't gotten around to it... 33% said they don't have enough assets to pass on to their loved ones, 13% said the estate-planning process is too costly, and 12% said they do not know how to get a will" (Konish, 2022).

That's a serious lack of planning! Everyone needs to make these decisions before they become necessary. And there are lots of necessary decisions to make. In Chapter 7, I'll talk more about your lasting legacy. But for now, I want to explore with you the nitty-gritty details of ensuring that your future plans encompass all the boring but essential factors that face you before your journey through life comes to a close.

Planning is especially important for the childless person who is getting older. You don't want circumstances to catch you unprepared. You'll need to make sure that you have financial plans in place and that you've got healthcare covered.

These decisions aren't ones to take lightly. They affect your life now and the lives of your loved ones later. It's better to avoid the complications that come with a lack of planning. It may sound totally daunting at first, but never fear. I'm here to guide you through the maze!

## Plan Your Future

Your wishes and your future are important, not just to you but to those around you. They affect you, it's true, but they also affect those you will inevitably leave behind you. I know that you want to make it easier on them as well as yourself. But that can only be assured if you start making arrangements now. A combination of educating yourself on financial matters and putting that knowledge to use is what you need.

You're used to making plans and decisions for all kinds of things—where and how you'll live, who you choose to let into your life, your work life from your first job to your chosen career, and especially your life without children. Those decisions become even more important now. But you have to consider the possibility that you're not going to be able to manage your own affairs throughout your whole life. At some point, you will likely need help. You'll need to prepare for that eventuality.

What are the pieces of your plan? It includes investment, which can help ensure that you have something to leave your eventual heirs. Then there's your retirement, which can hinge on your investment strategy. You also can't forget to plan your estate. Rest assured, however, that there are people who can help you with the whole process. Here's a quick guide to what you need to know.

## Making Investments

I've heard it said that investing in the stock market is a form of gambling, and in many ways, that's true. You put money in, and you never really know how much you're going to get back. If you're not careful, you can lose everything. The odds of winning change daily or more often. And if you just put money in once and let it ride, you can get a nasty surprise down the line. Still, investing—in the stock market or other places—is a good way to increase the funds you have to live on as well as the inheritance you leave behind.

One important thing to know before you invest is how you view risk vs. reward. If you want a high return on your investment, you sacrifice safety—the reward is higher, but so is the risk. If you're willing to accept a smaller return, it's more likely that the investment is a safer bet. Assets like fixed annuities and bonds provide stable income but at a low rate of return. Stocks and commodities can make you more money, but the risk of losing money is also greater. Only you can decide how risk-averse you are.

Be careful, though. Con artists know that you likely worry about whether your retirement savings are adequate, particularly when you're faced with high medical bills. Scammers frequently promote investments offering unrealistically high rates of return. Don't be fooled. As the saying goes, if it sounds too good to be true, it is. Take the time to check out the investment and the person offering it. You should be especially suspicious of phone calls and emails that come out of the blue recommending sure-fire opportunities with quick, guaranteed returns. If you have questions or problems with fraud, the Securities and Exchange Commission (SEC) Office of Investor Education and Advocacy is a great place to start.

## Options for Investing

Some people are nervous about making investments. It seems complicated, and there's always a chance that you could lose your money if you're not careful. But that's no reason to keep your money under your mattress or even in a single bank account. There are smarter investment strategies that will help you keep the money you have and add to it over the years. Here's a look at different ways you can invest your funds:

- **Cash**: Keep your cash in a high-yield savings account or money market account. Make sure they're covered by FDIC insurance. Your checking and savings account combined should cover four to eight months' expenses. One drawback to savings accounts is that inflation will mean that your rate of return is less than you anticipated. But savings and money market accounts are easy to draw funds out of for emergencies.

- **Stocks**, also called **equities**, are shares in a company that you can invest in. When the stock price goes up, you make money. On the other hand, when it goes down, you lose money. Diversification, or having investments in more than a single company, is a good idea—not putting all your eggs in one basket, so to speak.

🚶 **Bonds** are essentially loans that you make to a company or the government. The interest you receive is likely to be lower than that for stocks, but the returns are guaranteed. **Treasury bonds** are backed by the U.S. government. Here, you trade low rates of return for security. Seniors may want to keep half of their money in bonds.

🚶 A **Certificate of Deposit (CD)** is a type of savings account. Your money is tied up for a certain period of time, usually three months to five years, at a fixed rate of return. At the end of the term, you get your money back plus interest. That interest is generally higher than what a regular savings account yields. Withdrawing your money early brings a penalty.

🚶 An **annuity** is a contract you make with an insurance company. You deposit an amount of money, which draws interest. You get paid a fixed amount of income every month based on how much money you used to fund the annuity. An annuity can be a good supplement to your retirement income.

🚶 A **mutual fund** is a diversified combination of assets such as stocks, bonds, and other securities. Such funds can have different strategies, such as investing in larger or smaller companies. Money market mutual funds are a safe investment but don't yield large rewards.

- 🚶 **Commodities** are goods like gold, oil, or farm products that you invest in, hold for a certain amount of time, and then sell. Sometimes, people hold a commodity like gold physically. Commodities are good to buy before inflation hits, but of course, predicting when that will happen is difficult at best.

- 🚶 **Real estate** is another form of investment. You can own a building or buildings and rent them out to provide you with income. One version, called a Real Estate Investment Trust (REIT) is a company you can invest in that owns a variety of properties, such as warehouses, offices, and other commercial locations.

There are other types of investments, too, such as cryptocurrency and hedge funds. An investment professional can steer you toward the best ones for your age group and retirement status. The tax liability for each of these investments differs. Make sure you get an explanation from the financial institution or your financial advisor so the tax bite doesn't surprise you.

Which investment should you choose? Having a combination of several types, as well as cash, is a good way to achieve long-term success. One pro recommends, "One rough rule of thumb is that the percentage of your money invested in stocks should equal 110 minus your age, which [for someone 70 years old] would be 40%. The rest should be in bonds and cash" (Wolfson, 2023).

# Retirement

Most people retire sometime between the ages of 50 and 65. Of course, if you're able to retire sooner or choose to retire later than that, great! But either way, you need to make plans. Your retirement plans will depend on your particular circumstances. But whatever your situation, your retirement will require a good deal of budgeting and planning and, most likely, advice from a professional.

You can think of retirement as being divided into four phases: pre-retirement, early retirement, middle retirement, and late retirement. You'll have different needs during each of these phases and different strategies to employ as you move through them.

During the **pre-retirement** phase (ages 50–62), you need to start evaluating your likely needs and examining your resources. Is your mortgage paid off yet? What can you expect to get from a pension plan, Social Security, or other retirement plan such as a 401(k) or IRA? Can you take early retirement or a buyout from your employer? Do you need to increase your savings and investments? Do you need to consider staying in the workforce longer? Can you plan ways to reduce your spending or increase your income?

The **early retirement** phase encompasses ages 62-70. Sometime during that time span, you'll probably apply for Social Security. The longer you postpone doing that, the higher the monthly payment you receive will be. Social Security payments increase when the cost of living rises, but not necessarily enough to keep up with inflation. You'll also have to contend with the fact that you no longer have employer-sponsored health insurance. It's time to start shopping around or to save for expenses that Medicare won't cover.

In early retirement, you may also be able to take advantage of other sources of income. You can use the expertise you've developed throughout your career to start your own business, or you can take on part-time or seasonal work to supplement your income. You could take on "gig" or contract work in a field like copywriting or audio production for podcasts.

**Middle retirement** brings you to the ages of 70 to 80. At the age of 73, you are required to take at least minimum distributions from some of your tax-free retirement accounts, so you'll have that additional income. However, you may want to focus on cutting your expenses and saving some money every month. You might consider moving to a smaller house or apartment and renting out your current home, or perhaps one room or floor of it. Or you could potentially take in renters who would share your home with you and provide additional income.

After age 80, you move into the **late retirement** phase. One of your main concerns will be healthcare costs, especially those that Medicare doesn't cover. If you need to move to an assisted living facility or another sort of living arrangement, you will also incur increased expenses. Your other expenses are likely to remain the same as they were in middle retirement. One potential solution to increased expenses might be a reverse mortgage, a form of loan in which you draw out the value of your home, usually without making mortgage payments.

One option that may be open to you when you retire is to move to a location with a lower cost of living. If your job required you to live in New York City, Chicago, or another expensive place to live, when you're no longer working, you could move a distance from the city or even to a different state where you won't have to spend so much on housing, taxes, and other expenses.

A question many retirees have is whether their income will last until the end of their lives. Of course, there's no way to know exactly when that will be, but there is a handy rule of thumb that can help. Investment professionals recommend that you withdraw 4% to 5% of your investments each year and then adjust for inflation every year. If you have a rate of return of 6% on your portfolio, this will ensure that you don't tap the principal. This is known as the Safe Withdrawal Rate or SWR. It's not a guarantee that your money will last throughout your retirement, but it does limit the amount you withdraw so that your portfolio is better able to withstand economic downturns (Hayes, 2021).

As a childless individual or couple, retirement planning is different for you. While parents may find themselves "empty-nesters," their needs will still differ from yours. You may have spent more of your income on your own needs and wants instead of spending it on the many expenses of raising kids. Or you could have saved more of that "extra" income and have it available to you now. A couple with no children who saves $550 each month from age 30 to age 48 with a 7% rate of return would have over $200,000 of additional retirement funds. If they then let their investments grow and accumulate until age 70, they could have as much as $1,000,000 of additional retirement funds, which they can use for medical expenses, nursing home expenses, or other needs. The key is to start as soon as possible and to save and invest as much as you can afford (Gigante, 2021).

## Estate Planning

You don't have to be one of the super-wealthy to need an estate plan. Really, everyone should have one, and that goes double for people with no children. Unless you want the courts to decide what happens to your assets if you become incapacitated or pass away, you need to make arrangements in advance.

Why? You don't really want to let the courts make all the decisions, do you? Or have your assets become the property of the state? Estate planning is your best bet for avoiding these outcomes. In addition to making your wishes known, it will save your heirs a lot of trouble. It's estimated that "following a loved one's death, American families spend an average of 500 hours and $12,700 over the course of 13 months (20 months if probate is required) to finalize the person's affairs and settle their estate" (June, 2022). Dying without an estate plan can eat up many years and dollars, lose value due to federal and state taxes, and put your wishes in legal limbo.

What sorts of arrangements do you need to put in place? In addition to a will, you will need to consider at least one of the following—probably more than one:

- **Living will**: This document defines your wishes should you be incapacitated, such as whether you want to be resuscitated in the event of cardiac arrest.

- **Medical Power of Attorney**: Also called a health care proxy, this goes to someone who has the authority to make the same kind of medical decisions for you. This person will be an advocate for you if you are unable to make these decisions for yourself.

- **A trust** will hold title to your assets for the benefit of a third party. The person who holds the title is called the trustee. The beneficiary can be anyone you designate.

- **Financial Power of Attorney**: This important document allows someone to take care of your bills, taxes, business, Social Security, home, banking, and investments while you aren't able to look after them yourself. Your financial power of attorney doesn't have to be that of a lawyer. It can be a financial professional or someone you trust.

- **Life insurance**: Some people have a modest life insurance policy to cover their final expenses. Others have large policies that will replace their income for a beneficiary, such as a spouse or partner. Your life insurance policy—and some other investments, such as an IRA or 401(k)—will have you designate a beneficiary and a contingent beneficiary if the first person you choose is not available.

- **Information release**: This document, which could be supplied by a hospital or a lawyer, gives your doctor permission to inform a designated person about your medical condition.

- **Executor**: When you write your will, you will name an executor to oversee how your will is carried out, including matters such as taxes and debts. There are professional executors you can hire if your affairs are complicated. The cost might be up to 5% of your estate (Pitsker, 2018).

Childless seniors often choose a friend or family member to carry out their wishes as recorded in their living will and powers of attorney. But you should also name a backup person ("successor") in case your first choice isn't available or able to carry out the responsibilities.

## Advisors and Assets

The best advice regarding your finances is to find someone who can give you advice regarding your finances. You read that right! A financial advisor is the right person to guide you through the often-confusing decisions that need to be made to make your money work for you. But how do you find a financial advisor? And how do you make sure that the financial advice they give will really meet your needs?

First, you need to determine what your financial needs really are in order to decide who's the best person to help you. A financial advisor can work with you to maximize the returns on your investments. But they can also help you with regard to your retirement plans, debt repayment, tax planning, budgeting, and even your choice of insurance plans and products. You may not need all those kinds of advice, so you can choose an advisor who specializes in the areas you need the most help with. For example, since you don't have any children—and if you don't have much debt— you may want to employ an advisor who works mostly in the field of retirement planning.

You also need to know that there are few laws about who can call themselves financial advisors, so you need to make sure that the person you choose has your financial interests at heart. There are advisors who have what's called a "fiduciary duty" to you, which means, legally, they're required to give you advice that's in your best interests. Other advisors are only required to recommend products that are "suitable" for you, even more expensive ones, or ones that earn the advisor a higher commission.

Basically, there are four different kinds of financial advisors. Which one you choose depends on what you're willing to pay for:

- **Fee-Only Advisors** are paid based on the amount of resources they invest. They could also charge you a flat rate or an hourly fee. Because they get their money from you, they have fewer conflicts of interest.

- **Commission-Based Advisors** make their own money based on the products they sell you. One word of caution: These advisors may advertise their services as free because you don't pay them directly. They get their commissions from third parties.

- **Registered Investment Advisors** are usually large firms that are paid a yearly account fee or a percentage of what you invest. They have a wide range of expertise and are suitable for almost all of your financial arrangements.

- **Robo-Advisors,** as the name suggests, are automated investment platforms you find online. You pay a flat yearly or monthly fee, usually a comparatively low one, or an amount based on your assets. They're especially good for mid- to long-term investments, such as retirement planning.

If your needs are more for bookkeeping and tax matters, you might also consider working with an accountant.

## Choosing Your Advisor

Of course, you can ask your friends, peers, or financial institution for recommendations, and you can use an online search tool to find an advisor in your area, but there are ways you can determine for yourself whether a particular advisor is right for you.

First, do some research on the potential advisor's background and credentials. Professional advisors can be verified by the Certified Financial Analyst Institute or the Certified Financial Planners Board. Both have websites you can consult. An advisor may also specialize in a specific area of advice, such as retirement planning or the stock market.

Find an advisor you can communicate well with. This means not only that they have regular office hours and return your calls, but also that they use language you can easily understand rather than technical jargon. There are certain complex concepts that need to be addressed, but your advisor should be able to define and explain them.

There are also a number of questions you can ask a potential financial advisor to determine if they're a good fit for you and your needs:

- Is my first consultation appointment free of charge?
- How do you get paid—through fees, commissions, or bonuses for selling products?
- What services do you offer?
- Is there a minimum limit on the accounts you handle?
- What's your investment philosophy?
- How much will I pay for your services?
- Are you licensed or certified?
- How often will you communicate with me?
- Who will be working with me? You or another advisor?
- Will you collaborate with other advisors on their specialties?
- Do you conduct virtual meetings in addition to or instead of in-person ones?

## Safeguarding Your Assets

Choosing the right financial advisor is one key to protecting your assets against the time when you really need them. It's a devastating prospect to think that your carefully acquired assets might suddenly (or gradually) disappear due to fraud or other underhanded dealings. But choosing a reputable, effective financial advisor is only the first step. You also have to watch out for attempts to steal your financial information or even your identity. Identity theft is a particularly insidious crime. It can take years to recover from the damage it causes.

## Protection From Scams

I think by now we all know not to give our financial information or any money to Nigerian princes claiming to need help, but there are lots of other scams and trickery that can deplete your finances. The people behind them often target seniors, thinking that they're easy targets. You should make them regret that assumption! The scams often go unreported and are difficult to prosecute, though, so it's best to be on the lookout for fraud. They typically prey on emotions like fear or excitement.

One of the simplest scams is the phone call that starts with a simple "Can you hear me?" Your initial tendency will be to say, "Yes," but that's a mistake. Scammers can record your response and then use the "yes" to authorize purchases on your credit cards. In fact, you may want to avoid answering calls you don't recognize altogether. You can also cut down on nuisance calls by not answering your phone with "hello." That can trigger an automated system to put a person on the line who will pester you about buying some goods or services. It's smarter to answer with your name ("This is Louise") or some other phrase ("What is this in regard to?").

Other dangerous phone calls are those that say they're from the IRS or another government agency. None of these are legitimate. The IRS never contacts anyone by phone; they specialize in sending letters, often certified. The scammer is just trying to get your personal information, like your Social Security number, in order to steal your identity.

You could also get a call saying it's from a computer support department, stating that your computer has been compromised and that you need to pay to get it restored. A real computer company won't reach out to you this way. You have to contact *them* with problems. They could also ask to take control of your computer remotely. When they do, they can steal all kinds of private information. One way to combat these scammers is to ask for a phone number you can call them back at. At that point, they may well hang up on you. Or you can take great satisfaction in telling them you don't believe them and simply hanging up. Then, report them to the FBI's Internet Crime Complaint Center (IC3), the AARP Fraud Watch Network, or the Better Business Bureau.

Romance scams abound, too. If you engage in online dating or chatrooms, you can be vulnerable. They create fake profiles on social media so they appear legitimate and spend time softening you up. They may claim to be (or actually be) located overseas. Requests for money at first sound reasonable or urgent. Once you've given in to one request, the next one will be for a larger sum. When you realize you're being scammed or stop sending money, your romantic correspondent counts on you being too embarrassed to report the theft.

One good protection from various kinds of fraud is to set up credit card and bank account fraud alerts. The company will contact you if there is a transaction over an amount that you set, if there is a charge that wasn't signed for, or if one comes from an overseas or questionable source. Other companies provide stand-alone identity theft insurance and help recover your information and money. If you see suspicious charges on your statement, you may have to cancel your credit cards and get them replaced with new ones.

## Reflection

Consider what you have done so far to ensure your legal and financial future and what else you can do to improve your plans.

- Which of my legal and financial documents need updating?
- How confident am I about the effectiveness of my retirement plan?
- What professionals might help me fine-tune my plans?
- What investments can I choose that will suit my risk-reward profile?
- Am I prepared to protect my assets from fraud and theft?
- Who should hold my financial and healthcare proxies?
- Do I need to revise my retirement budget?

## Affirmations

Reinforce yourself for the knowledge and abilities you have that will serve you well in legal and financial planning.

- I am smart and capable.
- I make good decisions.
- I am in control of my future.
- I am looking forward to the future.

* I can take care of the people closest to me.

* I can increase and protect my assets.

## Coming up Next

Your legal and financial plans will ensure that you live well as you grow into your senior years. But you need to think about your physical well-being too. In the next chapter, I'll guide you through ways to keep your body healthy and strong.

# CHAPTER 6

# HEALTH AND LIVING ARRANGEMENTS

*Aging is not "lost youth" but a new stage of opportunity and strength.*

**–Betty Friedan**

Ben and Harriet never had children, and they revel in their lives together. But as they age, they encounter problems living without someone else to care for them. Fortunately, they are in good health, thanks to regular visits with Dr. Sefton, their primary care physician, who helps them deal with any illnesses, gives them advice on how to stay strong and healthy, and advises them on what they need to do to remain safe in their home.

The couple intends to stay in their own house as long as possible before they move into the senior care facility they chose. Harriet searches the internet for products that will help them avoid injuries, and Ben installs them. Together, they found an apartment that could be converted to meet their physical needs. Harriet uses a wheelchair, while Ben has arthritis in his hands and sometimes struggles with his balance. In particular, Harriet worried that Ben might fall in his home office or shower while she was away at work.

They modified their home to meet their needs. The bathroom includes features that reduce the possibility of falls. The kitchen was equipped with tools that Ben could easily use to cook and clean. They didn't need children to fuss over them and look after their health. Ben and Harriet were proud that they could manage themselves.

Many people who are getting older find that they need to pay careful attention to their health. They face unique challenges, from chronic conditions to the natural consequences of aging, including injuries and illnesses. They need a network of health professionals and a support system that can help them prevent or deal with physical difficulties or their effects.

Those who experience aging without children may have additional concerns about staying safe in their own homes or apartments. There are the dangers of falling and suffering injuries without someone there to help or call for assistance. Fortunately, seniors who live alone can adapt their homes to increase the possibility of ensuring safe and comfortable living.

## Staying Healthy

Getting healthy and staying healthy are the best solutions for many of these problems. Healthy living can extend your lifespan and make sure that you stay well enough to thoroughly enjoy your life. There are lots of aspects of health to consider, though. Here's some help in finding the best ways to ensure that you live long and happily:

## Healthy Living

You've all heard about the three most important aspects of good health: sleep, diet, and exercise. They're key throughout your life, but even more so when you're a senior.

## Sleep

Sleep is restorative for the body. Dreaming helps the brain process memories. And sleeping well is an integral part of maintaining good health. Unfortunately, many seniors experience sleep problems. Just like other adults, you need to get at least seven hours of sleep per night.

You may have trouble getting that much, though. Pain, getting up to urinate frequently, sleep apnea, restless legs syndrome, and plain old insomnia are some of the reasons you could be short on sleep. Sleeping pills, while they can help, bring problems of their own, including hallucinations, agitation, bizarre behaviors, memory problems, and even addiction. It's better to get sleep the natural way.

A number of techniques can help ensure you sleep well. Here are some dos and don'ts:

- Make sure that your bedroom is comfortable, including the room temperature as well as the bedding.

- Do keep a sleep schedule, going to bed and waking up at the same time each day.

- Develop a routine for just before bedtime. Relax with a warm bath or shower. Meditate if that is something you like to do. If exercise relaxes you, try not to do it right before you try to sleep, though.

- 🚶 Don't take long naps during the day or close to bedtime.

- 🚶 Don't use electronic devices near bedtime either—the blue light they put out will cause you trouble sleeping.

- 🚶 Don't have a nightcap at bedtime. Alcohol will cause sleep disruption.

## Diet

You know from years of experience that you need to eat a healthy diet full of fruits and vegetables, protein, fiber, vitamins, and minerals. But as you age, your eating habits may change. Your appetite could lessen. You may have difficulties because of mouth problems or dentures. Medication side effects can alter how food tastes and smells.

**Here are some dos and don'ts for healthy eating.**

- 🚶 Do take a multivitamin supplement, plus calcium and iron, as well as vitamins A, B12, C, and D.

- 🚶 Do get enough calories every day. Women 60+ need from 1,600 to 2,200 calories, and men 60+ need 2,000 to 2,600, depending on their level of physical activity.

- 🚶 Do ask your doctor about drug-food interactions. Grapefruit and other foods can make medications less effective.

- 🚶 Don't indulge in alcohol and smoking, which can make food taste blah.

- 🚶 Don't take chances with food-borne illnesses. Use proper food handling and sanitation.

🚶 Don't skip meals. You need to keep up your strength, and regular eating is key.

## Exercise

No one's saying that you need to be a bodybuilder or a triathlete (though it's great if you can be). But keeping yourself moving has benefits for your bones and muscles, as well as your flexibility, heart rate, blood pressure, stress level, and chronic conditions such as obesity. You can experiment with a number of forms of exercise until you find the one that's right for you. Here are some exercises you can try and some tips to make them more effective.

🚶 Yoga and other stretching exercises can be done even if you have movement limitations. You can enjoy the benefits of plenty of exercises using a chair or wall for balance.

🚶 Walking, biking, dancing, and swimming are great aerobic exercises. They're good for your heart. Just be sure to avoid high-impact aerobics like running, which can be hard on your joints.

🚶 Strength exercises such as weightlifting will help keep your muscles strong. Start with light weights and increase them as you gain strength. If you use a wheelchair, do arm exercises to keep them at peak performance.

🚶 Exercising at least three days per week is best, but any physical activity you engage in, such as yard work, will be good for you.

🚶 Warm-up and cool down before and after exercising to keep your muscles loose and flexible.

🚶 Stay hydrated. Even if you don't feel thirsty, drink water before, during, and after your workout.

## Your Healthcare Needs

What exactly do you need in the way of healthcare? You may not know unless you have an assessment of your requirements. The person to do that assessment is a gerontologist or geriatrician, a medical professional who specializes in the disorders that accompany aging. Their assessment will include your general physical well-being, your cognitive function, your nutrition, any illnesses or conditions you have, the medications you take, and even your social support system.

It used to be that people visited doctors only when they were ill or dying. Now, regular checkups are your best defense when it comes to monitoring your health and receiving preventive care. They allow you to find potential problems before they become more serious. Catching warning signs early makes diseases and disorders easier to treat. And that can reduce healthcare costs.

Because people differ in their health status, the assessment is designed to compare your chronological age with your "functional age," a measure of what you're able to do and what specific health concerns you may have. This assessment is more detailed than the usual tests and questionnaires that you usually get when you visit the doctor. It's an overall picture of you and how you're doing in terms of your health status.

The assessment will help your doctor develop a treatment plan. For example, if you report that you have had several falls in the past six months, your treatment plan will probably include some form of physical therapy to improve your balance.

You need to have tests, screenings, and other procedures as you age. For example, in your 50s, talk with your doctor about what screenings and tests they would recommend. As you enter your 60s, you should get eye exams, hearing tests, dental checkups, and a colonoscopy. Don't forget cancer screenings such as mammograms, as well as blood pressure and cholesterol tests. Various risk assessments and other screenings are also recommended: depression, fall risk, diabetes risk, and heart disease risk. Some risk assessments are available online. Your family history of various illnesses and conditions will also be important, so you may want to have a list of those handy.

And don't forget your flu, pneumonia, and COVID vaccines, and perhaps a shingles vaccine. In your 60s or 70s, have an osteoporosis risk assessment (if you haven't already had one by that time).

## Healthcare and Your Support Team

You'll probably need more than one doctor—medical personnel for a variety of age-related conditions. First of all, you need a primary care physician, an internal medicine doctor, and maybe a geriatrician for all your everyday illnesses and problems. Other specialists may be necessary as well, such as an oncologist, ophthalmologist, endocrinologist, rheumatologist, or orthopedist, depending on what your needs are. These people are your partners in health care, but you need to be an active participant too. After all, it's your health we're talking about!

How do you find providers to be part of your healthcare team? First, ask your primary care physician to refer you to a specialist. They will probably have a number of trustworthy providers they've worked with and can recommend. Next, contact your insurance company. They'll have a list of doctors in your area who specialize in various fields and who are part of your plan. This will limit your choices, especially regarding specialists. Make sure whoever you choose has privileges at your preferred hospital. Your insurance company may have a particular hospital or even a pharmacy they favor.

Your friends can make recommendations based on whom they see and trust. Schedule an appointment to see whether you feel a rapport with them and what your credentials are. You can also look up physicians on the internet and check out their credentials, specialties, and even reviews from their patients.

If you have depression or other mental or emotional problems, consider going to a therapist. You can select from a number of different practitioners. A psychiatrist may suggest that you see a psychologist who can prescribe medication. For a therapist, you can choose one who specializes in mood disorders or a particular kind of therapy, such as couples therapy or cognitive therapy. If you prefer, you can see a church counselor, a crisis management therapist, or a clinical social worker, depending on your needs.

Nurse practitioners, physicians' assistants, visiting nurses, and home healthcare aides can also be part of your healthcare team. They each have specific roles. With home healthcare aids, you may have some say in who provides your care, but nurse practitioners and physicians' assistants work out of your doctor's offices.

When choosing any kind of healthcare provider, consider where their office is located, whether their office has plenty of parking and handicapped parking spaces, the office hours and after-hours availability, and even the provider's bedside manner, attitude regarding newer medications and procedures, and—perhaps most important— whether the doctor treats you with respect and dignity. Being able to communicate openly with your provider is also important. Medicine is filled with large, unpronounceable words. Does your doctor explain what they mean or leave you in the dark? Do they discuss treatment options with you? And do you feel comfortable discussing potentially embarrassing symptoms with them?

Also, your doctors may belong to a healthcare group that offers various online services such as appointment reminders, test results, and even the ability to pay your co-pays electronically with your bank account or credit card. You can opt to use these resources or not, as you choose. A healthcare group can also be a source of medical care when your doctor is on vacation or otherwise not available.

Anyone has the potential to become ill and incapacitated. If you're in that situation, you need someone who can make decisions for you. And if you're aging without children or a spouse, it's even more important to have someone who knows what kind of medical care and treatment options you want. Consider carefully who that person will be. Designating who will hold your medical power of attorney is up to you. But if you can't find a suitable friend or relative who lives close by, whom should you choose? If there's no one in your circle who's appropriate, you may want to select someone who knows the local medical scene—perhaps a retired medical professional that your doctor recommends.

But you are the most important part of your healthcare team. Scheduling yearly checkups (or more often if required) and following up on appointments are key. If physical or occupational therapy is prescribed, make sure you go to them and do any home exercises the therapists recommend. Take your medications faithfully, and don't stop taking them until you run out. This is especially important for antibiotics. If you experience side effects you can't tolerate, speak to your doctor rather than just stopping the medication. Consider getting a pill caddy that reminds you of what to take each day and the time you should take them.

Learning about any disorders you have will aid in your diagnosis and treatment, but be careful about what you may find on the internet. Lots of the information there is very general, misleading, or just plain wrong. If you do search the net, try looking for reputable organizations like the National Institutes of Health, the National Institute on Aging, the Centers for Disease Control and Prevention, and MedlinePlus.gov. Sites with ".gov", ".edu," and ".org" URLs are almost always more reliable than ones with .com extensions.

## Alternative Solutions

Diana enjoys a healthy lifestyle, taking her dogs for long walks every day and avoiding drugs, alcohol, and tobacco. She believes strongly in psychic phenomena and communicating with nature. The idea of using traditional medical solutions just didn't seem like something she wanted.

Fortunately, Diana has access to other kinds of practitioners. She consults with a local expert on nutrition, who advises her on her diet, recommending vegan or macrobiotic eating and using vitamins and other supplements to ensure that she gets all the nutrients she needs. She goes to a massage therapist to treat tight muscles and a chiropractor to help with backaches. She consults with other types of healthcare practitioners on occasions when she needs help in other fields. Fortunately, the area she lives in offers a wide variety of alternative medical care.

Whether you have specific medical needs that haven't been addressed or you have intolerable side effects from your prescriptions, you may want to explore the other options that are available to you. Alternative or "complementary" medicine is a booming trend in the U.S. and around the world. (Complementary medicine refers to strategies that are used as adjuncts to conventional medicine.) Many alternatives are based on medical traditions from around the world, in particular, eastern countries and Native American practices.

While relying on plants can be hazardous if you don't know much about their chemistry or biology, some herbs, flowers, and roots have proven to be beneficial. St. John's wort, for example, is widely recognized as a treatment for depression, and willow bark makes a tea that can be used for pain relief. Valerian and chamomile are recommended for anxiety. It's best to consult with an expert on plant-based medicine and to inform your doctor of any herbal medicines you use, as they can have bad interactions with more traditional drugs.

Acupuncture is another kind of alternative treatment. Developed from Chinese medicine, it involves placing thin metal needles at various points on the body and then manipulating them by hand or using electricity. It's been found to be effective in many cases for relieving back and neck pain, headaches, migraines, and knee pain. It's also used to treat anxiety and stress. Acupuncture has become so accepted that it has even been used in hospitals.

Massage therapy is used for loosening tight muscles and increasing joint flexibility in nearly any body part as the therapist rubs and kneads the body or applies hot stones along the spine. A gentle massage results in relaxation, while a deep tissue ("Swedish") massage probes muscles deeper under the skin. Massage is also good for general relaxation and improved sleep. Professional massage therapists go through extensive training that makes them familiar with the bones and muscles of the body.

Yoga and meditation, while not strictly forms of medicine, are often used to address problems such as lack of flexibility and anxiety. Yoga involves moving the body into specific positions or a series of them. It's beneficial for joints and muscles as well as balance. It increases blood flow and calms the mind. Meditation also has a soothing effect and works to concentrate the mind and calm anxiety.

(Mindfulness, which I discussed in Chapter 4, is a practice related to meditation.)

Chiropractic treatment uses spinal manipulation, or "adjustments," to correct bone alignment problems and relieve pain. Chiropractic practitioners often treat people whose necks or backs have been injured, perhaps because of a car accident or fall. There are certain drawbacks to chiropractic treatment, including the possibility of increasing joint pain and function. Also, it may not be covered by insurance. Osteopathic medicine involves manipulating the musculoskeletal system too, but osteopaths can also practice traditional medicine, such as ordering tests and prescribing drugs.

Combinations of these approaches can be found in holistic medicine and naturopathy, which include herbs, massage, acupuncture, exercise, nutritional counseling, and other forms of treatment. Together, they make up what is called holistic medicine because it stresses the health of the entire body and mind. Homeopathy is probably best avoided since it doesn't have proven benefits and can lead you to forgo more effective treatments.

## Your Home Options

One of the questions that many or perhaps most seniors, especially those who are childless, have is where they should live. The answer to that question changes as you age, of course, but it's worth exploring before your needs change. For example, Delena was able to live alone in her own home. She occasionally had an aide who came in for light housekeeping. The county where she lived offered a special bus that took seniors and mobility-challenged people to doctor's appointments and the like.

One day, however, a strong wind caught Delena's door and knocked her to the ground. Her neighbor checked on her to see if she was injured. She was. The impact broke several bones in her face, and she had to go to the hospital for several weeks. When she was well enough to be released, she realized that she couldn't live alone anymore and moved into a nursing home. There, she enjoyed activities designed for her age group, trips to shopping centers, music and exercise opportunities, and more. There was even a small aviary on the grounds.

There are many different options for living arrangements. Here's a look at what you can choose from when the time is right.

First and foremost is aging in place—staying in your own home. That's desirable for as long as possible. It preserves independence and is more flexible and comfortable. You have all your possessions around you. You may want to move into a smaller house or an apartment because of the difficulty of keeping up a larger place. And you may have friends who can share a house with you and provide both an antidote to loneliness and help with chores, transportation, and other needs.

Speaking of apartments, you can choose to live in a senior-only community. They're required by law to require at least 80% of residents to be 55 or older. Many communities have an even higher proportion of senior residents. The benefits include the amenities you might find in any apartment complex, such as a clubhouse or a pool. There are also senior-specific apartment buildings that offer accessibility features such as wide doorways, grab bars, or a limited amount of stairs.

Another fairly independent choice is one called an "accessory dwelling unit," or ADU. These small houses or converted outbuildings, frequently known as "granny flats," may be possible if you have a relative, such as an aunt, uncle, niece, nephew, or cousin, who has a suitable space available. In this kind of living arrangement, help is close by if you need it.

You can also band together with fellow child-free seniors in the kind of co-housing situation featured on the famous TV show *Golden Girls*. It's another form of aging in place. Sharing a house provides companionship, emotional support, and assistance with the tasks of daily living. Plus, you can share the rent!

Continuing care retirement communities let you have as little or as much assistance as you need. You start by living independently in an apartment or duplex, then transition to a more supportive environment as needed. As you age, you can move into assisted living, memory care, and then advanced nursing care arrangements.

Generally, to be avoided as long as possible, nursing homes provide the most care for seniors—including help with bathing, medications, meals, and getting in and out of bed. The more you can afford, the more amenities they offer. There are drawbacks to nursing homes. You have to choose carefully, as many nursing homes are understaffed or undesirable for other reasons.

## Safety and Convenience at Home

If you are able to remain independent in your own home, there are safety considerations, so you can stay there as long as possible. For example, you want to ensure that you don't suffer dangerous falls.

Bathrooms are places where many falls happen. There are solutions, however, and many of them are retrofits that can be installed by you or by professionals. Walk-in tubs or showers are good options, perhaps with a built-in shower seat. (You could also purchase a separate shower seat.) Grab bars and rails are highly recommended to avert slipping and falls.

Wheelchair ramps are no doubt familiar to you, but you may have to have doors widened as well. A ramp can also be a good idea if you have other mobility challenges, like arthritic joints.

You've no doubt seen TV ads for devices to summon assistance if you do fall. A monitoring service responds if you press the button, and it sends help. One thing to remember—the device only helps if you wear it! Delena fell outdoors once when she was freeing a dog from a fence. She remained there until a repairman happened by, heard her, and summoned her neighbor. Her emergency pendant was hanging on the bedpost at the time.

And while you're living on your own, remember that there are many adaptive devices and solutions that can help you with independent living. There are kitchen utensils that help with tasks that are difficult for arthritic hands. Adaptive cleaning products and tools are available too. You can find solutions for daily tasks such as getting dressed or even peeling a hard-boiled egg. A quick Google search will find companies that specialize in these products.

## Reflection

Think about your health and your living arrangements, and consider both what you're experiencing today and what you're likely to experience in the future.

- Am I able to live alone at the moment? How long is this situation likely to last?

- What illnesses or accidents might affect my ability to live alone?

- Have I made plans for my future living arrangements and needs?

- Am I in denial about being able to continue living independently for the rest of my life?

- What resources can I call on to help me live alone as I age?

- Have I begun considering or researching alternative living arrangements?

- Is there anyone nearby I can rely on for help?

- Do I have inaccurate ideas about life in a retirement community, continuing care solution, or nursing home?

- What can I do to make it possible to live in my home longer?

## Affirmations

- 🚶 I can make good decisions.
- 🚶 I realize what my needs are.
- 🚶 I will live independently for as long as possible.
- 🚶 I adapt to the changes in my life.
- 🚶 I know what's best for me now and in the future.
- 🚶 Needing help is not a sign of weakness.
- 🚶 I am good at planning.

Use these questions and affirmations to examine your living situation and plan your future according to your needs. You can take control of that future and do what's best for you.

## Coming up Next

Your physical well-being is only one aspect of your life. Considering your emotional well-being is important as well. As you live your life, you can harness that emotional strength to determine what your legacy should be and how you can achieve it.

# CHAPTER 7

# EMOTIONAL WELL-BEING AND CREATING A LEGACY

*The purpose of life is to discover your gift. The work of life is to develop it. The meaning of life is to give your gift away.*

–David Viscott

Roger and his husband, Scott, had a good life. Now entering their 60s, they were settled into the house they had built together. They enjoyed spending time with Scott's great-nephews, but they also enjoyed going home by themselves afterward. Outwardly, Roger and Scott ought to have been entirely satisfied and happy.

But Roger was suffering from uncontrolled stress. After 19 years as a supervisor in a correctional facility, he had had enough of people. Roger longed to leave his job and spend more time at home. The stress he had been under led to physical problems—tension headaches and ulcers, as well as crippling depression—that made him feel run-down and achy. His mental health suffered, too. At times, he didn't care if he woke up in the morning.

Scott was worried about Roger and told him so. Roger resisted, claiming that he didn't need any help. But Scott got Roger's oldest friend to tell him that he was worried too. Eventually, when he hadn't slept for several days, Roger agreed to get help and see someone.

After getting professional help and a course of medication, Roger felt well enough to look for another job. He found one as a greeter in a local store, which supplemented his Social Security. He found that, when he wasn't in charge of other people, he could relax and enjoy it when the shoppers stopped to chat with him. Scott noticed the change in his mood at home, too.

## Find Peace and Joy

Roger found that his emotional state affected other areas of his life. When his emotional and mental health suffered, so did his physical health and his relationships. Once he got help, his problems cleared up. But it would have been better if Roger had realized earlier that he needed to address what he was feeling.

Emotional well-being is often overlooked when health is being discussed. But it's an essential part of your life and needs to be cared for. Like Roger, you can seek professional help for disturbances in your emotional life. It's good to take care of your emotional health before you get to that point, however.

Along with physical health, emotional well-being is a facet of overall wellness that shouldn't be overlooked. As you age without children, you need to look at your emotional wellness, especially if you live alone. Roger had Clark and other friends tell him when they thought his emotional health was suffering. But if you don't have that social support network around you, you may not recognize the effects until your emotional equilibrium is out of balance. (Take another look at Chapters 4 and 6 for more on social support and finding fulfillment.)

As you grow older, your potential for feeling satisfied increases. Your child-free status is another important source of internal well-being. Together, these factors prepare you for a life of peace and joy.

## Emotional Well-Being

Your emotional well-being is the sum of your internal feelings and how well you cope with them. It encompasses physical health and mental health and is intimately connected with both. After all, there's no separating your body from your brain. They're part of a set!

Emotional wellness isn't just about being happy all the time. That's not realistic. Emotional well-being does mean that you're in touch with your emotions. You acknowledge them and recognize their importance in your life. You stay aware of your emotional state and its effects on your mind and body.

Your emotions are as important as your intellect when it comes to addressing difficulties and facing challenges. You'll be better able to do that if you're not weighed down by fear and distress. Of course, fear and distress are natural emotions that you will feel at times, and you should be able to notice and acknowledge them.

But negative emotions have an important place in your life. They warn you when something is wrong. Roger felt anxiety and dissatisfaction when he needed to leave his job and look for more joy in his life. Fear tells you that you are facing some kind of threat. It makes you aware that there is something you need to deal with.

The problem is that your emotions are not used to modern problems. Fear and anxiety were useful when our ancestors faced danger from wild animals, for example. They were signals to fight or flee. Nowadays, however, these feelings arise when there are no physical threats. They still have the same effects on the body, which releases fight-or-flight hormones that raise your heart rate and blood pressure and tense your muscles to prepare for physical confrontation. If you live with anxiety and stress most of the time, the chemical changes in your body don't abate, and you're left with only the physical effects. Think about how your hands shake and you breathe heavily after you're threatened by a large, snarling dog. Your body doesn't realize that there's a fence between you and the threat.

With emotional well-being, you recognize when you are feeling stressed and do something about it. You do many of the same things to alleviate emotional and mental stress that you do when you want to remain physically healthy. As I discussed in the last chapter, sleep, diet, and exercise are vital to physical health, and they're key to emotional and mental health as well. For example, exercise releases "feel-good" chemicals that are effective in improving physical and emotional well-being. Think "runner's high," and you've got the idea.

Threats to mental health are a growing problem in society. It's estimated that one in five Americans will have some form of mental or emotional difficulty in their lifetime. Anxiety and depression are found throughout society, thanks to the fast pace of modern society, the stresses of work, and fears for safety. The recent COVID pandemic, in particular, affected many people in ways that made them feel helpless. Because they were cut off from their usual sources of emotional support, they didn't have the opportunity to talk out their problems. And because many were cooped up at home with family, tensions between them increased.

## Nurture Your Emotional and Mental Health

Being in touch with your emotions isn't the only way to help ensure emotional balance. There are many techniques that you can use to achieve and maintain balance in your life. Try these suggestions to take care of your mental and emotional needs.

- Once you're aware of your emotions, find ways to express them effectively. If you're annoyed by a coworker, for example, don't fly off the handle. Tell them what's bothering you without getting angry. Let yourself calm down before you address the problem. When you're not so agitated, say, "I feel disappointed that you didn't get the sales figures to me on time." Then, tell them how to address the problem—"Please get them to me by the end of the day." There. You've expressed how you're feeling *and* suggested a way to solve the problem.

🚶 Maintain a healthy work-life balance. (Of course, this is easier to do if you're retired.) Set boundaries around your time. For example, draw a line with your boss about being available by phone or text after business hours. If you're the boss, set a boundary for yourself that you won't take work home on the weekends or stay up late at night working. Allow yourself time off and a chance to enjoy your personal time or time with your significant other.

🚶 Focus on the positive in your life. It's not realistic to turn every negative into a positive. Sometimes, bad things and unpleasant feelings happen, and it's best to recognize them and deal with them instead of ignoring them or denying they exist. But when you feel unsettled or dissatisfied, remind yourself of the positive aspects of your life, such as the activities you enjoy, the special people in your life, your religious faith, the fact that you're in good physical health, or whatever else you appreciate.

🚶 Along that line, use your reflection journal to record your positive feelings. Another way to reinforce positive feelings is to keep a gratitude journal, either as part of your feelings journal or a separate one. Take pictures of things that bring you joy—pets, vacations, your spouse or partner, outings with friends, your softball team—and keep them in your journal. Use them as wallpaper on your phone, tablet, or computer.

🚶 Even a short time outdoors can help you get rid of a bad mood and relieve stress. A walk in the fresh air and sunshine or a quick game of tennis provides an opportunity to get away from your problems and restore your spirit.

- 🚶 Consider getting a pet. The act of caring for another living being can improve the way you feel. A wagging tail or a purr is something to enjoy and savor. Can interacting with a pet relieve stress? Maybe. The scientific jury's still out on that, but lots of pet owners find it to be true.

- 🚶 Use technology to relieve stress, not cause it. Look for calming apps such as nature sounds, videos that guide you through meditation, or blogs that focus on positivity. Limit your screen time, especially at bedtime. But if it relaxes you, you can occupy your brain with online puzzles or games. They can keep your brain busy without overthinking or entertaining unpleasant thoughts.

- 🚶 Give yourself a treat! It doesn't have to be a diet-busting goodie. Occasional pampering will give you a lift. Of course, it's not going to provide emotional balance all by itself, but a spa day with a relaxing massage or a day trip to a nearby destination can revitalize you.

But if none of these techniques work well enough to alleviate your stress and calm your emotions, you can—and should—look for other forms of help. Some problems are just too complicated to handle alone. Remember that you have options. Therapy or medication (or both) could really aid you in recovering your emotional balance. Don't wait too long. If you find yourself asking whether you need to seek help, you probably do.

## A Routine to Foster Emotional Balance

When you think "routine," you think boring, dull, and lifeless. It sounds crazy, however, but it's true—routine is not the enemy of a healthy emotional life. It's the basis for it. Keeping to a daily routine grounds you. It provides the framework for a healthy life and a calm, productive brain.

You already know that regular meals and daily exercise are two keys to physical health. They're also important for maintaining emotional well-being. When you get into the habit of having a nutritious meal at the same time every day, you have something to look forward to. It's the same with exercise. At first, it may seem like a chore and a bore, but before long, you'll find yourself getting into the groove of daily stretching, jogging, or whatever your favorite form of exercise is.

Your brain needs exercise, too, and you can find an opportunity to keep it active every day. The daily crossword or sudoku puzzle is one way to get your gray matter revved up in the morning. Or you can read for an hour every evening before it's time for bed, soaking up knowledge on a nonfiction topic or giving your brain a challenge with a twisty whodunnit mystery.

Daily meditation is a good form of relaxation or a spiritual boost. Allow yourself a time for meditation when you first get home from work so you can unwind and refresh. Or start your day with a centering meditation to prepare you for what's ahead. As you continue with the practice, you'll find that it becomes an indispensable part of your day. If prayer or reading a daily devotion is part of your spiritual practice, making it a daily priority will help you maintain a feeling of calm and connectedness.

Schedule some time each day for social interaction, even if it's just answering your email and texts. Contact with the world outside is vital for your emotional health. Or you can schedule a regular weekly breakfast date or chess game with your partner or a close friend. That'll get you out of the house as well, which can be a break from your usual routine or an essential part of it.

If you play an instrument or are learning a new language, daily practice will improve your performance. When you set a regular time for it, you'll soon start noticing real improvement, bringing you increased satisfaction and positive feedback that is good for your emotional well-being.

Don't skip regular appointments and activities. That haircut, volunteer work at the animal shelter, or after-work drink with your buddies can be the thing that lifts your mood or helps you put your worries on hold for a while.

The bottom line: You don't want to get into a rut, but a varied routine of self-care and engagement with the world will do wonders for your emotional and mental health. Scheduling your life-affirming activities means that you won't neglect your body, brain, and spirit.

## Leave a Mark on the World

Growing older without children can make you think about what kind of mark you will leave on the world. All of us want to be remembered positively. It's a universal desire. You want to believe that your life has meant something to the people in your life, your community, or the world. Having that kind of lasting impact means you will not be forgotten and that your life has meaning. It's an ambitious thing to want, but it's within your grasp.

You aren't being egotistical or grandiose when you think about leaving a legacy. A life well lived *should* affect the world in some way. The wisdom you've accumulated; the friends you've made; the contributions you've made; and your gifts of time, service, and financial support—all are part of your lasting legacy.

Now, while you're still active and vital, is the time to think about what your legacy will be. You still have time to make your mark on the world.

## Your Legacy

What is a legacy? It's a way for the world to remember you were here, a continuation of the good things you've brought to life. It's more than the material goods that you leave to your heirs. A legacy is an inheritance for the world. It's a way to touch other people's lives even after you've finished yours. In fact, "one of the most commonly expressed wishes among seniors was a yearning to leave a legacy... 75% of respondents said that it was important for them to be able to pass along their *values and life lessons*" (*How Seniors Can Leave a Legacy*, 2018).

There are also some advantages that childless seniors have when it comes to leaving a legacy. When you think about your financial legacies, you have a greater ability to make varied bequests because there's no expectation that you will leave the bulk of your assets to your children. Of course, you can leave any amount to other relatives: contribute to a retirement account or a college fund for a niece or nephew, for example. But your friends or your favorite charity can receive the bulk of your estate without causing a family feud.

## A Non-Financial Legacy

Perhaps just as important, though, is what you have to contribute to the world in terms of other assets than material goods. You have a lot of life experience that's valuable and worth passing on. And that's worth more than money in a very real sense.

You have the benefits of your education to share. You have the inspirations and passions that you have expressed throughout your life. You could well be the person who has been most responsible for keeping the family history intact. You can pass the extended family's documents along to the family members or members in the best place to continue to maintain and add to them. If you've kept up your correspondence with them, you have even more to share.

You have intangible assets to pass along as well. Chief among these are gifts of wisdom. Throughout your life, you may have been mentoring younger members of your extended family in their chosen careers or interests. All along, you've been enriching them with your time, attention, and knowledge. You've shared with them in many nonmaterial ways, especially spending time with them and fostering their passions as well as sharing yours. You've given gifts by demonstrating your ability to communicate your honesty and inspiration.

Your journals can be a rich resource for passing along your wisdom to others. You may not want to bequeath the ones that reveal your most personal thoughts, or you might consider these the most valuable assets you can possibly share. It's best to think about these matters before you make any formal arrangements so your heirs know what you want to do with them.

You can also use your assets to fund a different sort of legacy. As noted in Chapter 5, you have a variety of options: an annuity, trust, or other financial instrument that will benefit a cause, organization, or charity. Choosing a worthy recipient and helping to finance their work is a terrific way to carry on your values.

Then, too, you can leave some of your material assets to organizations where they'll do the most good. If you have a car, for example, you can leave it at a vocational school for student mechanics to learn. If you have created or purchased art, there may be a local museum that would value it. Or you could donate artwork to an organization that can auction the pieces to raise money for their cause. Even material possessions can be used for this purpose. One example is a musician who donates a fine guitar to be auctioned in order to provide funds for music lessons for underserved young people.

## Find Personal Fulfillment

Throughout your life, you've been able to express your innermost values and inspirations. When you're thinking about the legacy you'll leave, it's time to assess how you've fulfilled your personal aspirations. Is there anything you've dreamed of doing that you haven't accomplished yet? Now is the time to get busy with it.

It's not too late—it's never too late! Everyone's heard the example of the famous artists' Grandma Moses, who didn't start painting until she was 78, and Georgia O'Keefe, who remained vital and creative well into her 80s. Their lives are testimony that genius knows no age.

If there's any ambition that you haven't yet fulfilled, by all means, start in on it. Or if you've started an endeavor in the past but gotten away from it, know that you can pick it up again and continue your work. Tap into the creativity that has grown within you over the years. Chase that dream! Whether you finish or not—whether you finish that book you've wanted to write, have the gallery show you've dreamed of, or have built that independent consulting career—this is not the time to stop. It's time to renew your efforts.

Keep in mind, though, that in finding personal fulfillment, you should look at what you've already accomplished. Not everything you've started has been left unfinished. You have a wealth of experiences that you can truly treasure. There's the work you've done, the pleasures you've enjoyed, the education you've received, the friends you've made, the wisdom you've shared, the things you've created, the wealth you've earned, and the progress you've made toward your goals. All of those are accomplishments you can look back on and be proud of.

Some of the things you've found fulfillment in have been material, while others are less physical. Personal fulfillment is made up of a combination of the physical, the mental, and the spiritual. You may give greater emphasis to one over the others, or you may try to keep them in balance. Those are your choices based on your values and your passions. No one can say whether your choices are right or wrong. Choices are individual to the person, and yours are valid.

You have built your life through everything you've done, thought, loved, cherished, and devoted yourself to. You have created your life and your legacy in the best way you could. At times, it hasn't been easy, but you have persevered. That's an accomplishment in and of itself. You deserve to be proud of your accomplishment and the effort you've put into it.

In the end, your life is your testament to your passions and your posterity.

## Reflection

Throughout this chapter, I've encouraged you to examine your life—your past and your future, what you've done, and what remains for you to do. You've had a chance to reflect on what you want to be remembered for. Here are some questions that will help you with this process:

- What brings me peace and joy in my daily life?
- What has brought me peace and joy throughout my life?
- How have I fostered my emotional well-being?
- Do I have a daily routine that improves my emotional health?
- How do I want to be remembered?
- What steps can I take to make sure I'm remembered that way?
- Which of my qualities have I shared with others?

- What kind of legacy can I leave for my community?
- What values have been most important to me?
- How have I expressed those values throughout my life?
- What do I still want to accomplish?

## Affirmations

Take this opportunity to reinforce your pride in your accomplishments and your ambitions for the future. Take in these affirmations and repeat them to yourself, either silently or aloud. Let them sink into your mind and spirit. Let them guide you through your meditations on your life and legacy.

- I make choices that bring peace and joy into my life.
- I have a great capacity for feeling joy and fulfillment.
- I deserve to feel fulfilled.
- I can improve my emotional well-being.
- I have much to offer the world.
- What I have accomplished is a worthy legacy.
- I can still add to my legacy.
- My contributions improve my life, family, and community.
- I'm proud of how I've lived.

## What's Next

Congratulations! You've completed your journey with me through the facts and feelings of life as a senior without children. Now, it's your turn to continue the journey on your own. As you do, remember the things I've told you. The most important thing, of course, is that your life and your choices are valid. Also key is the idea that you've got a lot more life to live and that you can fill every moment of it with peace, joy, and fulfillment. Finally, celebrate your child-free life of wisdom and continuing satisfaction. You deserve it!

# CONCLUSION

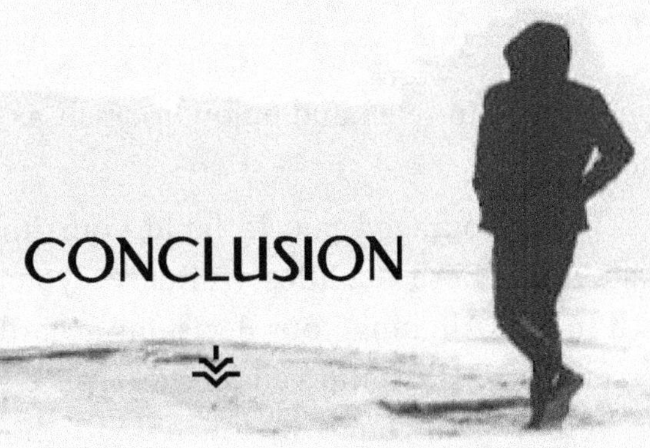

Congratulations! You've now been introduced to the positive aspects of growing older without children! It's a joyful journey if you take it step by step, treasuring your freedom and building your awesome life. I hope this book has helped you discover how you can embrace life as a child-free senior and provided answers to some of the questions and concerns you may have.

Within the pages of this book, I've offered validation for the life choices you've made. They're both valid and right for you—don't let anyone tell you differently! Now that you're a senior, you can reflect on those choices and what they've meant for you through the years and what they'll mean for the years to come. I know they'll be filled with even more reasons to celebrate the way you live and how you approach the rest of your life.

Despite the societal pressures that encourage parenthood, you have chosen another way: Living child-free. Whatever you've decided, you have good reasons that reflect your personal situation and values. And regardless of the fact that you face certain challenges in the years to come, you can feel satisfied that you have also tapped into the many benefits that come with living without children. Your burdens are in many ways lighter, and you have the opportunity to relax and enjoy yourself as you grow in age and wisdom.

I've encouraged you to build your inner strength and resilience. Those qualities will serve you well along your path in life. Aligning your decisions according to your own personal strengths and values will ensure that they're right for you. When you're in touch with the things that are important to you, you will find that your life is more fulfilling. Building a resilient mindset is possible if you employ the strategies I've explained. Resilience is a combination of self-awareness and mental agility. You face life's problems with the knowledge that you have it within you to persevere. Your emotions reinforce your purpose in life, and your heart and brain work together to get you to the point where you have confidence and pride in your abilities.

You can nurture that emotional strength by practicing self-compassion. Look at your emotions regarding growing older with no children. They may be confused at first. Then, treat yourself with the same kindness that you would show to a close friend. Become aware of your self-talk—your inner voice—and don't believe it when it tries to blame or shame you. You deserve to have a clear mind and steady emotions.

Remember that you don't have to have family close by to maintain the social connections that are so vital to your stability and contentment. You can find people who offer help and support all around you: at work, in your neighborhood, at your place of worship, or in clubs and activities you pursue. In-person interactions can be supplemented by harnessing the power of electronics to maintain your connection with friends and family who don't live near you. If you find you need help coping with your feelings, you can even get in touch with a support group or therapist. They can be an important part of your extended support system.

Joy is an important part of life, and you can achieve it if you pursue your passions. Think about the little things that make you happy and expand on them. Explore activities that you've always wanted to try but never have. Develop new hobbies or rediscover old ones that have fallen by the wayside. You can take your time as you contemplate new activities. If you want to travel, for example, you could have a great time learning about different destinations before you settle on one. Build up gradually to that bucket list trip with day trips to scenic local spots or locations within your state. Find a travel companion who can share your experience with you. Or investigate the possibilities that come with group travel. That's one way to make friends who share your interests.

Don't forget the many volunteer opportunities within your own community. They'll appreciate the help, and you can feel good about making a difference. You can find peace and contentment by attending to spiritual matters. A group that practices a religion that appeals to you can provide companionship as well as being uplifting. Or you can find fulfillment through solo practices that help you explore your own form of spirituality. Mindfulness and meditation can be good for your spiritual awareness as well.

When it comes to finances, child-free seniors have a lot to consider. There's the overall necessity of planning for your future. You don't want to run out of money while you're still going strong! Planning is the solution.

Planning for your retirement is made up of a number of components. The first is the standard retirement options that you may have in place, such as a company pension or retirement plan and your savings. However, these may not be enough. You can consider investing your money, and not just in the stock market. There are a variety of investment opportunities that range all the way from mutual funds, cash, real estate, and annuities to gold and other commodities. You have more freedom to decide on a number of different living arrangements, too.

There are also decisions to make when it comes to legal matters. Do you have a living will and a health care proxy? How about a financial proxy? All of these can be vital parts of ensuring your retirement years go smoothly. Have you made a will for disbursing your assets? Do you have advisors who can help you figure out the complexities? And do you know how to protect your assets against financial predators? You'll need to find answers to all these questions, and the advice in this book has led you to the right path.

Then, too, you want to stay healthy as you grow older. I've shared with you information on diet, sleep, and exercise that will keep you fit through the years. I've also given you tips on the tests and treatments you may need in your senior years. Remember that you can also choose alternative practitioners to supplement your healthcare. You can—and should—build a team of experts who can guide you through the maze of decisions you must make. But remember that you are the most important person in ensuring your future health. The decisions and choices are yours!

You also have choices when it comes to where to live. As a child-free senior, you have many different options, including living solo for as long as you can, moving to a locale with a lower cost of living, sharing a home or renting out rooms in a large residence, senior-friendly apartment communities, and, perhaps eventually, an assisted living facility. The decisions are yours. They weren't made for you by any children!

In addition to your physical health, you need to consider your mental and emotional health and well-being. Taking care of these aspects of your life will help ensure that your life is filled with peace and joy. That's important when facing difficulties and challenges. An important part of lessening stress and improving your satisfaction is maintaining a good work-life balance. If you can avoid bringing your daily cares home with you and find ways to relax your body and spirit, you'll be well on your way to a calm, enjoyable life. A routine that combines meaningful work, social interaction, mental exercise, hobbies and interests, relaxation, and occasional treats "just because" will perk up your mood and keep it that way.

And keep in mind that your personal fulfillment is the most valuable aspect of your life as a child-free senior. You can find that fulfillment by considering your strengths, values, talents, and desires and making them an important part of your life. Do the things you've always wanted to do. Your personal fulfillment is the best expression of the choices you've made throughout your life—and the ones you still have to make in the future.

As you navigate your senior years, you should also think about what you want to leave behind. Your legacy can mean financial support for relatives, but it can also include bequests to charities and causes you care about to help perpetuate your involvement with their important work. And don't forget the gifts of your wisdom and attention that you can leave for the future. Write a book, create art, keep a journal, or just spend time with friends and young relatives to pass along your knowledge and ensure that your personality will not be forgotten.

Nathan and Morena Jackson are a prime example of a childless senior couple. In their mid-60s, they have already lived a full and fulfilling life and have no desire to stop now. They have a circle of friends they treasure and spend time bowling and hiking. They attend chamber music concerts and practice the violin and viola themselves. Nathan and his partner live on their own in a two-story house, so they have a second floor they can easily rent out to a college student to watch their house when they travel and supplement their income.

Morena works with a local food bank and shares her business knowledge at a mentoring program for the tech-minded. Nathan paints in his spare time and jogs daily to keep his heart healthy. Together, they love to grow both flowers and vegetables in their garden. The vegetables come in handy as they also love to cook healthy meals for themselves and their next-door neighbors, Mark and Sabrina McCarty, who are an important part of their support system. The Jacksons and the McCartys are competitive in their weekly games of euchre and Trivial Pursuit. Sometimes, they go out together on what they call a "double date" for dinner and a movie.

Like the Jacksons and the McCartys, you too can build a beautiful life that will sustain you throughout your senior years. Rest assured that your choices regarding not having children won't prevent you from having love, involvement, and satisfaction throughout your life.

I wish all of you peace and joy!

# Chapter "Good Will"

## Your Chance to Inspire

You have the power to make a huge impact on someone else's life and help them step towards a future of true fulfillment. All it takes is a few words.

Simply by sharing your honest opinion of this book and a little about your own story, you'll show new readers where they can find all the guidance they need to set forth on the path toward their best life.

Helping others without expectation of anything in return has been proven to lead to increased happiness and satisfaction in life.

I would love to give you the chance to experience that same feeling during your reading or listening experience today...

All it takes is a few moments of your time to answer one simple question:

*Would you make a difference in the life of someone you've never met—without spending any money or seeking recognition for your good will?*

If so, then here is my small request from you again.

If you've found value in your reading or listening experience today, I humbly ask that you take a brief moment right now to leave an honest review of this book. It won't cost you anything but 30 seconds of your time—just a few seconds to share your thoughts with others.

Your voice can go a long way in helping someone else find the same inspiration and knowledge that you have.

Are you familiar with leaving a review for an Audible, Kindle, or e-reader book? If so, it's simple:

If you're on **Audible**: just hit the three dots in the top right of your device, click rate & review, then leave a few sentences about the book along with your star rating.

If you're reading on **Kindle** or an e-reader, simply scroll to the last page of the book and swipe up—the review should prompt from there.

# ABOUT THE AUTHOR

In *Journeying Alone, Journeying Strong: Aging Without Children*, Chrío Zoë presents a compassionate and illuminating perspective on a growing demographic facing the complexities and intricacies of aging alone. She delves into the challenges and triumphs of those who have charted their later years without the presence of children or conventional familial support networks. Drawing from a wealth of personal stories, scholarly research, and her own deep understanding of the aging process, Chrío Zoë sheds light on the emotional, logistical, and societal aspects of this often-overlooked journey. She hopes that this book will serve as a reassuring and enlightening companion for those on this unique journey, offering valuable insights and practical wisdom on aging with grace, resilience, and dignity.

Chrío has a knack for capturing the essence of life's complexities, intricacies, and universal truths through her writing, often presenting thought-provoking perspectives on various aspects of existence. Her life books are characterized by rich character development, as the author skillfully weaves together the stories of diverse topics, illuminating journeys, challenges, and triumphs. Through books, the author explores themes such as love, passion, victory, identity, personal growth, and the search for meaning, offering readers profound insights and moments of introspection.

Beyond Chrío's professional accomplishments, she also has a rich and multifaceted life outside of publishing. This book is a testament to her commitment to providing valuable insights and practical guidance. The author's books are often praised for their ability to evoke empathy in readers, fostering a deep connection between the readers and the valuable insights they encounter within the pages.

Chrío is a distinguished authority in various fields of study, bringing a wealth of knowledge and experience to her thought-provoking non-fiction works. As you delve into Zoë's manuscripts, you can expect to embark on an intellectual journey guided by Zoë's profound insights and intentional thought-provoking passion for self - development. Her non-fiction works continue to push the boundaries of knowledge, inviting readers to expand their horizons and gain a deeper understanding of life and its impact on our success.

Chrío's works have been praised for their meticulous research, insightful analysis, and the way they challenge readers to think critically about the world around them.

## Any one of Zoë's latest books....

### 1. Unlocking Infinity: Master the Art of Longevity

Learn How to, Boost Your Brain Health, Recharge Your Immune System and Restore Youthful Balance in 3 Easy Steps

## 2. Living Your Best Life: Radiate from Within

Ultimate Guide to Finding Purpose & Fulfillment in 3 Easy Steps.

## 3. Redefining Aging: The Art of Living Alone

How to Find Joy in Independence, Live Fearlessly & Maintain Longevity

## 4. Longevity: The Art of Aging Backwards

Step-by-Step Guide to Renew, Restore and Reverse Aging Mentally, Physically & Spiritually

## 5. The Positivity Code: Supercharge Your Life with Positive Thinking

Learn The Art of Positive Thinking, Changing Your Life One Thought at a Time

## 6. Alone, But Not Lonely: Aging on Your Terms

A Roadmap for Aging Independently, Striking Balance & Finding Purpose

## 7. Mastering the Steps to Success: Achieving Success at Every Rung

Proven Strategies for Overcoming Obstacles and Reaching Greatness. Develop, Learn, Succeed

**8. The Growth Mindset Code: Cracking the Secrets to Success**

Comprehensive Guide to Breaking Limits with A Growth Mindset, Cultivating Unlimited Possibilities

**9. The Superfood Prescription: Refuel Your Mind & Body**

100 Supercharged Foods to Revitalize & Transform Your Health

... is another testament to her dedication to delivering enlightening and captivating non-fiction literature. Whether you're a seasoned reader of non-fiction or new to the genre Zoë's work is sure to engage, inform, and inspire.

To stay updated on **Zoë Publishing's** latest projects and musings, visit us on **facebook.com/zoepublishing** and follow us on Instagram & Tik Tok **(@zoepublishing)**

# REFERENCES

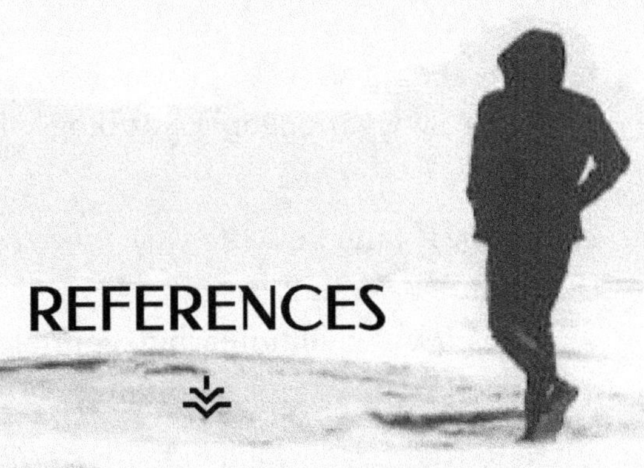


Adegoke, F. (2022, March 11). *The real reason Christopher Walken never had any kids.* The Blast. https://theblast.com/190737/the-real-reason-christopher-walken-never-had-any-kids/

*Aging Quotes.* (n.d.). BrainyQuote. https://www.brainyquote.com/topics/aging-quotes

*Benefits of mindfulness.* (2019, March 21). HelpGuide.org. https://www.helpguide.org/harvard/benefits-of-mindfulness.htm

Bertone, H., & Hoshaw, C. (2021, October 20). *Which type of meditation is right for you?* Healthline. https://www.healthline.com/health/mental-health/types-of-meditation#What-meditation-is-all-about

Birkin, R. (2020, May 5). *100 affirmations and mantras for fertility.* Robyn Birkin | Infertility Life Coach and Mind Body Practitioner. https://robynbirkin.com/affirmations-for-fertility/

Brown, D. (2020, April 2). *5 steps to building your spiritual practice.* Chopra. https://chopra.com/articles/5-steps-to-building-your-spiritual-practice

*Build a support system with a great network of people.* (2020, February 13). University of the People.

https://www.uopeople.edu/blog/what-is-a-support-system/

Burger, E. (2021, June 2). *4 life-enriching reasons to volunteer.* VolunteerHub. https://www.volunteerhub.com/blog/4-life-enriching-reasons-to-volunteer/

Cemental, R. (n.d.). *How to help seniors protect their assets.* Caring Senior Service. Retrieved October 18, 2023, from https://www.caringseniorservice.com/blog/protect-senior-assets

*Choosing the right doctor for seniors.* (2020, March 13). New Wave Home Care. https://www.newwavehomecare.com/choosing-the-right-doctor-for-seniors/

Clark, A. (2023, May 17). *Six safe investments for seniors in 2022.* The Senior List. https://www.theseniorlist.com/elder-law/investing/

Daniels, G. (2022, December 6). *The importance of leaving a legacy and how you can do it by example.* LinkedIn. https://www.linkedin.com/pulse/importance-leaving-legacy-how-you-can-do-example-glenn-daniels-ii/

Das, S. (2019, December 16). *15 awesome reasons to be childfree and not burden the earth anymore.* Bonobology.com. https://www.bonobology.com/awesome-reasons-childfree/

Delagran, L. (n.d.). *Why is spirituality important?* Taking charge of your health & wellbeing.

https://www.takingcharge.csh.umn.edu/why-spirituality-important

DeSilva, D. (2021, July 20). *Nutrition as we age: Healthy eating with the dietary guidelines.* Health.gov. https://health.gov/news/202107/nutrition-we-age-healthy-eating-dietary-guidelines

Eads, A. (2023, January 11). *How to find your passion for a more fulfilling career.* Indeed Career Guide. https://www.indeed.com/career-advice/finding-a-job/how-to-find-your-passion

*Emotional wellness: Its importance & how to make it better.* (2020, October 1). BioNeurix. https://bioneurix.com/blogs/blog/importance-of-emotional-wellness

Erieau, C. (2019, February 20). *The 50 best resilience quotes.* Driven App. https://home.hellodriven.com/articles/the-50-best-resilience-quotes/

*Financial planning quotes (89 quotes).* (n.d.). Www.goodreads.com. Retrieved October 4, 2023, from https://www.goodreads.com/quotes/tag/financial-planning?page=3

*Finding a health care provider for seniors.* (2023, July 21). Blog.providence.org. https://blog.providence.org/blog/what-to-look-for-in-a-senior-health-provider

*Finding hope and happiness beyond childlessness.* (2023, March 17). Kashmir Observer.

https://kashmirobserver.net/2023/03/17/finding-hope-and-happiness-beyond-childlessness/

*5 reasons emotional wellbeing is crucial for older adults.* (2020, February 11). Home Care Assistance Tampa Bay. https://www.homecareassistancetampabay.com/why-is-strong-emotional-health-crucial-for-aging-adults/#:~:text=Emotional%20wellbeing%20also%20plays%20a

Fontinelle, A. (2023, July 25). *Budgeting for the 4 financial phases of retirement.* Investopedia. https://www.investopedia.com/articles/personal-finance/110315/4-phases-retirement-and-how-budget-them.asp

Frost, R. (1915). *The road not taken.* Poetry Foundation; Poetry Foundation. https://www.poetryfoundation.org/poems/44272/the-road-not-taken

Fuscaldo, D. (2021, May 30). *4 reasons estate planning is so important.* Investopedia. https://www.investopedia.com/articles/wealth-management/122915/4-reasons-estate-planning-so-important.asp

Gigante, S. (2021). *How to set a retirement savings plan for DINKs.* Mass Mutual. https://blog.massmutual.com/retiring-investing/dinks-savings-plan

*A guide for seniors: Protect yourself against investment fraud.* (n.d.). https://www.sec.gov/files/guideforseniors.pdf

Ha, J.-Y., & Ban, S.-H. (2020). Effect of resilience on infertile couples' quality of life: an actor–partner interdependence model approach. *Health and Quality of Life Outcomes, 18*(1). https://doi.org/10.1186/s12955-020-01550-6

Hayes, A. (2021, November 27). *Safe withdrawal rate (SWR) method: Calculations and limitations.* Investopedia. https://www.investopedia.com/terms/s/safe-withdrawal-rate-swr-method.asp#:~:text=The%204%25%20rule%20states%20that

*Healthy eating, nutrition, and diet.* (n.d.). National Institute on Aging. https://www.nia.nih.gov/health/topics/healthy-eating-nutrition-and-diet

Hicks, C. (2021). *How to find a financial advisor if you're not rich.* U.S. News & World Report. https://money.usnews.com/financial-advisors/articles/how-to-find-a-financial-advisor-if-youre-not-rich

Hood, J. (2020, February 3). *The benefits and importance of a support system.* Highland Springs. https://highlandspringsclinic.org/the-benefits-and-importance-of-a-support-system/

*How older adults can get started with exercise.* (n.d.). National Institute on Aging. https://www.nia.nih.gov/health/how-older-adults-can-get-started-exercise#activity

*How seniors can leave a legacy.* (2018, May 24). Sagewood. https://www.sagewoodlcs.com/blog/seniors-can-leave-legacy-marketplace-wisdom/

*How to find reliable health information online.* (2023, January 12). National Institute on Aging. https://www.nia.nih.gov/health/how-find-reliable-health-information-online

Huddleston, C. (2023, January 23). *How to protect your finances as you age.* Getcarefull. https://getcarefull.com/articles/how-to-protect-your-finances-as-you-age

*Importance of identifying your strengths and weaknesses.* (2022, September 30). Make Me Better. https://www.makemebetter.net/importance-of-identifying-your-strengths-and-weaknesses/

*The importance of regular check-ups.* (2017, April 7). Pomona Valley Health Centers. https://mypvhc.com/importance-regular-check-ups/

*Involuntary childlessness.* (n.d.). COPE. https://www.cope.org.au/planning-a-family/happening/involuntary-childlessness/

June, A. (2022, June 20). *3 reasons why single folks with no children need an estate plan.* Www.linkedin.com. https://www.linkedin.com/pulse/3-reasons-why-single-folks-children-need-estate-plan-amy-june/?trk=pulse-article

Katz, A. (2014, November 19). *6 steps to invite spirituality into your life every day.* Mindbodygreen. https://www.mindbodygreen.com/articles/how-to-invite-spirituality-into-your-life-every-day

Konish, L. (2022, April 11). *67% of Americans have no estate plan, survey finds. Here's how to get started on one.* CNBC. https://www.cnbc.com/2022/04/11/67percent-of-americans-have-no-estate-plan-heres-how-to-get-started-on-one.html

Krähenbühl, M. (2022, February 21). *Childlessness is on the rise.* OpenEdition Books; Graduate Institute Publications. https://books.openedition.org/iheid/8864?lang=en

Lagemann, J. (2022, September 30). *11 meaningful ways older adults can volunteer right now.* Forbes Health. https://www.forbes.com/health/healthy-aging/volunteer-opportunities-for-older-adults/

Lambert, G. (2023, February 22). *How to protect your assets from a lawsuit or creditors.* Investopedia. https://www.investopedia.com/articles/retirement/07/buildawall.asp

*Manage your health in your 50s.* (2019, October 12). Www.healthdirect.gov.au. https://www.healthdirect.gov.au/manage-your-health-in-your-50s

*Manage your health in your 60s.* (2019, October 12). Healthdirect.gov.au; Healthdirect Australia. https://www.healthdirect.gov.au/manage-your-health-in-your-60s

*Manage your health in your 70s and older.* (2020, February 5). Www.healthdirect.gov.au. https://www.healthdirect.gov.au/manage-your-health-in-your-70s-and-older

*Mental health: Keeping your emotional health.* (2000, May 1). Familydoctor.org. https://familydoctor.org/mental-health-keeping-your-emotional-health/#:~:text=Emotional%20health%20is%20an%20important

Meyer, C. (2022, May 13). *9 best senior travel groups to join for an epic adventure.* Second Wind Movement. https://secondwindmovement.com/senior-travel-groups/

Natale, N. (2021, April 14). *Dolly Parton says she never had kids because she made "sacrifices" for her career.* Prevention. https://www.prevention.com/sex/relationships/a29992912/does-dolly-parton-have-kids/

Newsom, R. (2022, March 18). *Aging and sleep: How does growing old affect sleep?* Sleep Foundation. https://www.sleepfoundation.org/aging-and-sleep

Orlando, E. (2021, March 4). *Positive affirmations for infertility.* Infertile Millennial. https://www.infertilemillennial.com/post/positive-affirmations-for-infertility

Pitsker, K. (2018, June 7). *Planning for retirement as a single person.* Kiplinger.com. https://www.kiplinger.com/article/retirement/t047-c000-s002-planning-for-retirement-as-a-single-person.html

*Rediscover you: 10 benefits of solo travel over 50.* (2023, June 9). CORR Travel. https://www.corrtravel.com/10-benefits-of-solo-travel-over-50/

Rosenblatt, C. (2023, March 26). *Essentials for the solo ager.* Forbes. https://www.forbes.com/sites/carolynrosenblatt/2023/03/26/essentials-for-the-solo-ager/?sh=6084271a77c0

Samuels, C. (2023, June 23). *Senior isolation facts.* Www.aplaceformom.com. https://www.aplaceformom.com/senior-living-data/articles/senior-isolation-facts

Sayings, F. Q. &. (n.d.). *Top 59 quotes about childless: Famous quotes & sayings about childless.* Quotestats.com. Retrieved October 4, 2023, from https://quotestats.com/topic/quotes-about-childless/

Schmidt, J. (2023, October 17). *How to choose a financial advisor.* Forbes. https://www.forbes.com/advisor/investing/how-to-choose-a-financial-advisor/#:~:text=Ask%20friends%2C%20family%20and%20peers

Schoch, D. (2022, November 18). *Senior housing options.* https://Www.helpguide.org. https://www.helpguide.org/articles/alzheimers-dementia-aging/senior-housing.htm

Schweitzer, S. (2023, April 11). *The benefits of volunteering.* Northern Virginia Family Service. https://www.nvfs.org/the-benefits-of-volunteering/#:~:text=Volunteering%20is%20an%20enriching%20experience

Scott, E. (2023, April 27). *What is spirituality?* Verywell Mind. https://www.verywellmind.com/how-spirituality-can-benefit-mental-and-physical-health-3144807

*7 steps to leaving a lasting legacy.* (n.d.). Tonyrobbins.com. https://www.tonyrobbins.com/business/how-to-leave-a-legacy/

Stein, S. (2023, February 24). *11 reasons people choose not to have children.* Psychology Today. https://www.psychologytoday.com/us/blog/what-the-wild-things-are/202302/11-reasons-people-choose-not-to-have-children#:~:text=Some%20people%20feel%20they%20cannot

Sudhanshu, S. (2021, April 29). *6 hobbies elderly can pursue post-retirement.* Eldr—a Lifestyle Platform for Elders. https://eldr.co/lifestyle/hobbies/6-hobbies-elderly-can-pursue-post-retirement/#:~:text=According%20to%20a%20study%2C%20playing

Sutevski, D. (2021, October 1). *Elderly safety tips: Money and assets.* Entrepreneurship in a Box. https://www.entrepreneurshipinabox.com/27435/elderly-safety-tips-money-and-assets/

Sweatt, L. (2016, December 8). *11 Quotes about leaving a legacy.* SUCCESS. https://www.success.com/11-quotes-about-leaving-a-legacy/#:~:text=%E2%80%9CYour%20story%20is%20the%20greatest

*10 mindfulness activities for seniors in retirement.* (2021, June 8). Heritage Woods – Senior Retirement Communities Winston-Salem, NC. https://www.heritagewoodsseniorliving.com/10-mindfulness-activities-for-seniors-in-retirement/

*30+ tips for smoother senior travel.* (2019, July 23). Greatseniorliving.com. https://www.greatseniorliving.com/articles/senior-travel

Todd, B. (2021, March). *How to identify your personal strengths.* 80,000 Hours. https://80000hours.org/articles/personal-strengths/

*TOP 25 support systems quotes (of 97).* (n.d.). A-Z Quotes. https://www.azquotes.com/quotes/topics/support-systems.html

US Census Bureau. (2021, December 14). *Childless older adults more educated, more likely to live alone than older parents.* Census.gov. https://www.census.gov/library/stories/2021/12/no-kids-no-care-childlessness-among-older-americans.html

Walker, E. (2011). *Are there disadvantages to being childfree?* Psychology Today. https://www.psychologytoday.com/us/blog/complete-without-kids/201105/are-there-disadvantages-being-childfree

Walker, E. (2012). *Advantages and disadvantages of being childfree.* Psychology Today. https://www.psychologytoday.com/us/blog/comple

te-without-kids/201204/advantages-and-disadvantages-being-childfree

Waterman, G. (2022, July 7). *The top 5 financial scams targeting older adults.* Www.ncoa.org. https://www.ncoa.org/article/top-5-financial-scams-targeting-older-adults

Waters, S. (2022, July 11). *How to develop a resilient mindset: Recovering from setbacks.* Www.betterup.com. https://www.betterup.com/blog/resilient-mindset

*What is a geriatric assessment?* (2022, February 18). Cancer.net. https://www.cancer.net/navigating-cancer-care/adults-65/what-geriatric-assessment#:~:text=A%20geriatric%20assessment%20is%20a

*What is estate planning, and why is it important?* (n.d.). Www.nationwide.com. https://www.nationwide.com/lc/resources/investing-and-retirement/articles/what-is-estate-planning

*What is it like to grow old without any children?* (n.d.). Quora. Retrieved October 9, 2023, from https://www.quora.com/What-is-it-like-to-grow-old-without-any-children

Wolfson, A. (2023, March 15). *I'm 70 and weighing whether to "sell everything" and put it all in Treasuries, or hire a financial adviser even though it would cost $20K a year. What should I do?* MarketWatch. https://www.marketwatch.com/picks/im-70-and-weighing-whether-to-sell-everything-and-put-it-all-in-treasuries-or-hire-a-financial-adviser-even-though-it-would-cost-20k-a-year-what-should-i-do-

6793bfba#:~:text=Indeed%2C%20a%20good%20mix%20of

Wood, S. (2015, July 27). *12 practical ways to kick-start your daily spiritual practice*. Sumaiya Wood. https://sumaiyawood.com/kick-start-your-daily-spiritual-practice/